Whose Spine is it Anyway?

Wendy Emberson has been working in private practice since 1980. She left the NHS in order to give her patients the time, specialist clinical expertise and advice that she felt her patients deserved.

This book is the first in a series of nine that includes all the advice and tips that she has provided for her patients (and students) over the last 37 years in particular.

This series will offer the same approach, but to all the other areas of the body in turn.

Wendy Emberson MCSP
Stort Physio Ltd
Jenkins Lane
Bishop's Stortford
Hertfordshire
CM22 7QL
www.stortphysio.com

To my family, staff and patients for all their help and understanding.

Contents

CHAPTER 1 — 1

THE PROBLEM — 1

CHAPTER 2 — 11

THE STORY OF BACK PAIN — 11

CHAPTER 3 — 27

THE BACK EXAMINATION — 27

CHAPTER 4 — 59

THE DIAGNOSIS — 59

CHAPTER 5 — 76

TREATMENT FOR LOW BACK PAIN — 76

CHAPTER 6 — 92

WHY IS POSTURE IMPORTANT? — 92

CHAPTER 7 — 97

MEDICATION — 97

CHAPTER 8 — 100

NOW LET'S HAVE A SERIOUS LOOK AT ARTHRITIS — 100

CHAPTER 9	**103**
FEAR AND ANXIETY	103
CHAPTER 10	**107**
PAIN	107
CURRENT PAIN CONCEPTS	109
FOR PEOPLE WITH ACUTE OR SUB ACUTE PAIN	117
CHAPTER 11	**122**
DOs & DON'Ts OF BACK CARE	122
CHAPTER 12	**133**
EXERCISES	133
HOW TO HELP YOURSELF	133
A FINAL WORD	**140**

Chapter 1

THE PROBLEM

1. In any one year, in industrialised countries, up to half of the adult population will experience low back pain.
2. It is estimated that 4 out of every 5 adults will experience back pain at least once in their lives.
3. Back pain is just as common in adolescents as adults.
4. Back pain starts in school children and peaks in adults between 35 - 55 years of age.
5. The total cost corresponds to between 1% and 2% of the gross national product.

The NHS spends more than £1 billion per year on back related costs including:

1. £512 million hospital costs.
2. £141 million on GP consultations.
3. £150.6 million on physiotherapy treatments.
4. £565 million in the private sector.

£1.6 billion is the total healthcare costs for back pain in the UK, in addition to:

£590 - £624 million additional indirect costs to employers.
On any one day, 1% of the working population are on sick leave due to back pain[1].

These are huge costs and yet:

90% will get better within six weeks

---

[1] Figures from www.backcare.org.uk

A very important point here is:

7% of people with low back pain account for 90% of the health care costs

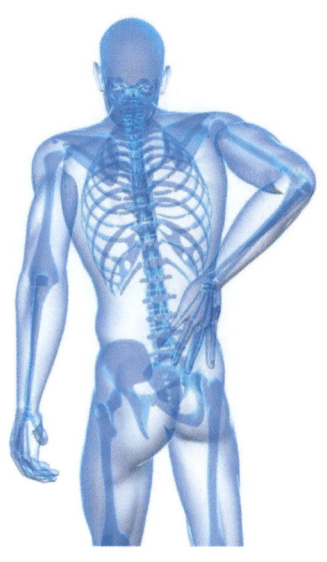

WHY?

It is my experience that people with so-called "simple low back pain" get very little information, or the right treatment necessary to prevent them from developing into chronic low back pain sufferers with all the attendant costs to them as individuals, and to the country.

Simple low back pain is not fashionable or newsworthy. Why? Because it is not life threatening and most people get it!

This book is for the 90% of people whose back pain apparently clears up in the six weeks with little or no treatment - to stop you becoming part of the 7%.

With the right information, then you can take the control and the responsibility for your own well being. As physiotherapists, we work WITH the patient instead of just doing something TO them. We need to move away from the idea that "a pill" or "an operation" will answer all of man's ills.

It seems to me that there is a lot of similarity with our education system! In schools, most of the effort is put into the super bright and the children with special needs. The great "grey masses" in the middle, the "average" children, are largely allowed to muddle through on their own! This is so short sighted!

If we put more effort into the so-called "average" low back pain patient, then we could have a much fitter population in every sense of the word. We need to balance the equation of costs and effort.

My work, as a musculo-skeletal (MSK) physiotherapist, is to prevent acute problems becoming chronic ones and to give you the knowledge and understanding of the problem of low back pain, how to deal with it and how to avoid it in the future.

There are so many healthcare practitioners, books, adverts and advice on the market today that all claim to have a cure for back pain. If any one of them lived up to their claims then surely the entire medical profession, NHS and all insurance companies would be providing it and very few people would have low back pain. After all, low back pain is not generally a life-threatening condition, but it does cost an inordinate amount of money to every western country, let alone the personal cost to the individual sufferers.

Interestingly the incidence of low back pain has not increased over the last 25 years or so, but the cost has increased by over 2000%

Why is this? One aspect may be that more people are claiming sickness benefit where most people will have just got on with it in the past. Also the cost of medication prescribed by GPs has increased, and maybe more people are claiming long term disability benefit.

It's not going to be a simple financial/medical equation as low back pain has become a significant multifaceted problem.

So why am I writing this book to add to the great mass of information out there that seems to do nothing but confuse everybody? Simple answer is that I want to give you the benefit of my training, postgraduate courses and observations over the 41 years that I have been a chartered physiotherapist.

During that time I have treated more patients with spinal problems than anything else. This amounts to seeing many thousands of patients presenting with a whole range of symptoms with the title of "non-specific lower back pain".

My specialist postgraduate knowledge and experience is in the very specific area of musculoskeletal medicine that used to be known as Orthopaedic Medicine. It was originally developed by Dr James Cyriax.

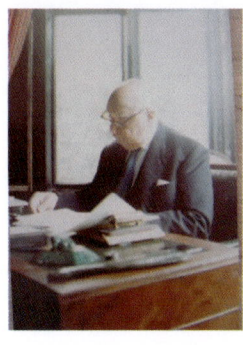

He spent 50 years of his working life identifying a vast number of conditions that can affect the musculoskeletal system *that you can't see on X ray*.

He developed a diagnostic and clinical examination system that is still unrivalled in the world today and even the latest scans such as MRI and dynamic ultrasound scanning are not as accurate as Dr Cyriax' system. It is a point worth noting that scans are only as good as the person reporting on them!

We now know that not all pain has a tissue-based origin. We know far more about pain than we did at the time when Dr Cyriax was working and we know far more about the physiological mechanisms of chronic pain as opposed to acute pain. Pain mechanisms are complex and we do not yet know the full answers as to why some people can have a simple acute problem which resolves quickly and easily, and yet others develop a pain mechanism that can go on for years. I will deal with this in a later chapter.

This is where I consider the problems start.

In my opinion, the reason we have such a persistent epidemic of low back pain is really down to the poor diagnosis and management of low back pain. Dr Cyriax' system is not taught routinely to medical or physiotherapy students. It is offered as an extensive postgraduate course, usually spread over two years, to allow for clinical practice between the courses. There is an examination at the end which can then lead to a Masters degree in musculoskeletal medicine.

This course needs to be offered at post graduate level as it needs the palpation and interpersonal skills, together with examination, treatment skills and knowledge etc that only comes with seeing and treating patients over a number of years.

One of the other major issues is that generally speaking, the medical profession prefer to use tests that gives them numbers or pictures. Something they can record, look at and compare. Medicine has advanced enormously over the last hundred years and especially over the last 50 years.

The technology involved in providing these numbers and pictures is truly incredible, but it is focused on the activity of the cells in the human body and their reaction to injury, disease or response to medication etc. I fully understand and appreciate the need for tests that are specific, measurable and repeatable. What we have learned from these tests about illness and disease is undoubtedly remarkable, even though we have some miles to go yet in searching for effective treatment as opposed to just management strategies.

This approach to finding answers to disease processes is completely laudable in constantly searching for how to prolong life. But that is only one aspect of our lives as human beings.

Of course we all want to live longer, but only if we can stay reasonably fit, in body and mind, to do the things we want to. The thought of reaching 80+ with a functioning mind, but a body that doesn't work, fills me with dread.

The other way round is an equally unpleasant prospect. So, full power and credit to the doctors and medical researchers who are working so hard to find answers to the life-threatening conditions and those working to find answers to the disabling neurological diseases.

What is not generally considered to be important by the medical profession is actually how the body moves, and how we can carry out complex movements and actions in a macro, rather than micro sense. Problems of the musculoskeletal system are not exciting because there is no threat to life. There is also little peer recognition of finding an answer to problems that will affect us all, but not kill us off!

The other issue is that the medical profession has but two approaches to problems:

1. Chemical warfare via medication.
2. Cut out the offending bit with surgery.

I fully appreciate that this is obviously gross simplification of two areas that demand great knowledge and expertise and it is amazing the results that can be achieved with these approaches.

The problem is that most people, including the medical profession, consider that anything that does not include drugs and surgery cannot possibly be of any value to the human condition. **All other forms of treatment are considered to be secondary to the main thrust of medicine today.**

In the treatment of disease that may well be true, but you cannot remove the person at the centre of this endeavour - the patient who is suffering the condition.

The diagnosis and treatment of low back pain can be a minefield and I want to give you just a few of the histories I have been told during my 4 decades of work as a clinical physiotherapist. From these examples, I hope you will understand why I have written chapters about the clinical examination process that I believe every patient with low back pain should expect and receive.

MISSED RARE, BUT SERIOUS PATHOLOGY

A 40 year old man came to see me complaining of pain in the thoracic spine (between the shoulder blades). On close questioning the pain had started about a month before, but in his low back and leg. There was no history of an injury or accident. It had just started one day as a low back ache and pain in one leg. It steadily worked its way up the spine to where it became acutely painful between the shoulder blades. He had seen an osteopath when the pain was only in his low back and leg. He went to his GP when it became obvious that the pain was getting worse and not better and his GP referred him to a consultant who in turn referred him to me.

I was not happy with this history of a progressive pain that involved more than one spinal level, and after a detailed examination, I referred him back to the consultant who reluctantly saw him again.

Within 2 months, this young man had died of septicaemia. What was eventually found was that the urethra (the tube from the kidneys to the bladder) had a weakness in the tube wall at one point. This meant that is started to balloon as it filled with urine, which in turn caused pressure on the nerves coming out from the spine. As the "balloon" got bigger, it put more and more pressure on more and more nerves. Unfortunately, this very rare condition was found too late and the "balloon" burst, spreading urine into his abdomen and causing the septicaemia.

*The lesson here was that a pain that progressed to include more than one spinal level ie in the back, down the leg **and** up the spine, should have been taken very seriously. 3 health professionals missed this fact by only taking part of the history. This may well have been through lack of available time to see and examine him, and it was a very rare situation, but if a few more particular questions had been asked, then this man may still be alive today.*

JUST ONE OF THE FAULTS IN THE SYSTEM

One patient more recently, came to see me complaining of acute low back pain, which had subsequently progressed to acute sciatic pain in the leg. At that point, the history and the examination did not raise any immediate concerns, but she was in a serious amount of pain from what was coming from damage to the last disc in the spine. This disc material had pressed onto her spinal cord causing the initial low back pain and then had shifted slightly to one side causing the pain in the leg – the sciatica.

This is a more common presentation, but I was concerned about the level of the pain she was experiencing in a short space of time. I treated her very conservatively using Interferential Therapy (see Chapter 5) to reduce the pain and inflammation in her low back and sciatic nerve. I also warned her of a possible complication where it can be possible for there to be a loss of control in passing water or faeces, and that this must be taken very seriously if this should happen to her.

She came back the next day and reported that she was beginning to lose control when passing water and that she felt she was losing some muscle power in her leg.

I immediately wrote a letter for her GP and rang the surgery to say that I wanted her to be seen that day. The GP saw her and tried to get her admitted to hospital as an urgent case, but the hospital would not see her on the recommendation of a GP. In the end, she paid to see the Consultant Orthopaedic surgeon at the local private hospital, who wrote a letter for her to take to Accident and Emergency Department. This was a letter referring her to himself in the NHS!

She was seen by the Consultant the next day and admitted into the local NHS hospital. The very necessary surgery was carried out just in time, before these symptoms had a chance to worsen and become permanent.

This is not such a rare situation and again I want to make sure that patients understand what is going on if certain symptoms arise that need urgent medical intervention. These are known as "red flags" and are covered in Chapters 3 and 4.

*What I find unacceptable is where patients can suffer irreparably harm, because the current system does not acknowledge that there are times when some patients need to be "fast tracked" through to Consultants. The knowledge and experience of health professionals working **outside** of the hospital environment are not see, or respected, as knowing when patients may be in urgent need.*

DON'T MISS THE BLINDINGLY OBVIOUS

Going to the other end of the scale, is the patient seen by a physiotherapy colleague. Admittedly, this case was not one about low back pain, but it does highlight very well the need not to miss the blindingly obvious!

The patient had an 18 month history of severe headaches, that only happened at night. He had been seen by three neurologists who were convinced that he had a brain tumour, but they couldn't find it on any scans.

He went to see this physiotherapist who asked him how he slept at night. He said he slept on his front, with five pillows! Without any treatment, she suggested that he should try sleeping on his back, or side, but with only 2 pillows to start with and to then try and reduce that down to one pillow. This he did and the headaches disappeared! No further "treatment" was needed. She applied the common sense approach in asking where did the "tumour" go during the day?

How much did that 18 months of investigations etc cost the NHS? That apparently simple question would have saved even more than just the money, it would have saved that patient 18 months of fear and anxiety thinking that he was about to die of a brain tumour.

ACCURATE DIAGNOSIS.

This patient had a history of nearly 2 years of low abdominal pain on one side only. She was referred by a consultant who had investigated everything internal and could find no reason for the pain.

A detailed clinical examination showed a marked problem with the sacro-iliac joints and there were no Red Flag issues (These are clinical signs that there may be serious pathology that needs referral to a consultant surgeon for example. See Chapter 3 for more detail). I asked her what had happened before this pain started, such as any accidents, slips, slides or falls and she said she had not suffered any of these. So I treated what was in fact quite a serious biomechanical problem with the joints in the pelvis between the sacrum, which sits at the bottom of the spine and the bones of the pelvis. One manipulation for these joints, Interferential Therapy and the start of a Recovery Programme and she was feeling a lot better.

The second time she came for treatment she told me how her daughter had reminded her that just before the onset of the pain, she had gone up into the loft and one foot had gone through the ceiling. This meant that the side of the trapdoor had struck her, quite forcibly, up between her legs and hit her on the bones of the pelvis. She had forgotten this episode as she just had a small amount of bruising and didn't need to go to hospital. She was sore for a few days and thought no more about it.

Within three sessions she had no pain at all and this was obviously the source of her pain.

The consultant in question had the good sense to refer this patient when it became clear that there was no internal cause for the symptoms. He had admitted that this was outside of his particular scope of practice and was happy to refer to someone who might have the answer. It is a great pity that this attitude is not more widespread. From the patient's perspective, it really needs all the members of the entire "healthcare professional team" to be fully aware of the different areas of expertise and when to refer to the appropriate specialist.

As physiotherapists, we are very aware of when to refer patients for consultant opinions. In other words, when a patient is not for us, but in general we cannot refer directly to a consultant and have to send the patient to their GP with our recommendation for a further referral. This can be very time

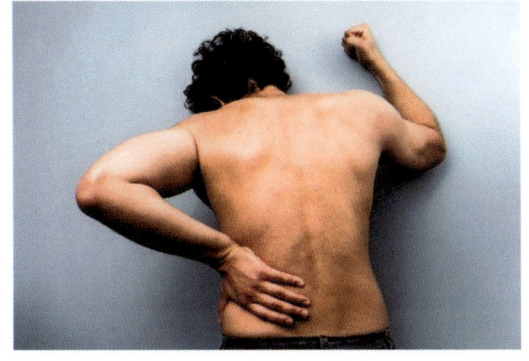

consuming for the patient and, as described above, may cause serious problems from the delay.

Chapter 2

THE STORY OF BACK PAIN

There is no doubt that low back pain is a problem that majorly affects Western, so-called First world, countries. Why is this?

IMPORTANT POINT

Less than 1% of low back pain is caused by a serious pathology or disease

BUT - Never before in the history of mankind, have so many sat for so long

There is no question that we all sit far too much these days. Even more when writing a book!

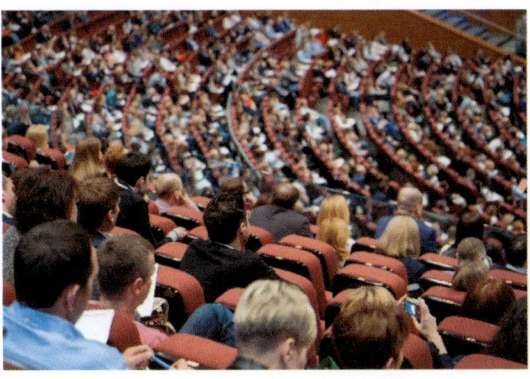

The problem is that we are not designed to sit on our buttocks/bottoms. The reason for this is that the sciatic nerve, which comes off at the last two vertebrae of the spine and the sacrum, passes through the buttock and under the bones in the bottom that we actually sit on.

At this point, the sciatic nerve is as thick as your thumb and it is the biggest nerve in the body. Yet we insist on sitting on it and squashing it between the bone of the bottom and the chair seat.

Few of us like sitting on a hard wood or plastic seat for any length of time and what we prefer is soft settees and sofas that have little support for backs and don't put too much pressure on our bottoms and sciatic nerves. That way we can last through a whole TV programme and maybe even the adverts without needing to shift weight or move! This is *not* a way to avoid low back pain, but it does avoid undue pressure on the sciatic nerve.

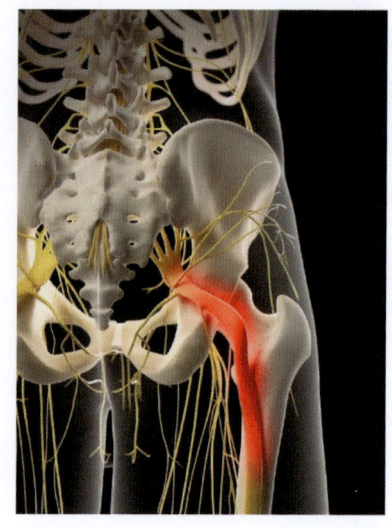

How many hours of your waking day do you spend sitting? I worked out that the average teenager spends only about 3 hours of a day actually on their feet!

As we get older, the time spent sitting at computers, or in cars/trains travelling to and from work, gets more and more. In this busy, hectic world we live in, we get home and sit again to eat and relax in front of the television.

Of course there are active people in the community, but the great majority spend far too long sitting - and generally sitting badly. What this means is that the body doesn't move very much and the soft tissues and joints accommodate to these patterns of movement. So, as we get older our joint ranges reduce and we end up doing less and less.

Africa, Asia and the Far Eastern countries will be travelling down our "low back pain road" as they follow our example in life style i.e. sitting more and more at computers and doing less and less physical activity.

China has about 80% less hip replacement surgery than we do in the UK, but the numbers are increasing. They will also start developing the back pain levels that we have as the population changes its life style to the Western model.

Some years ago, I was interviewed on the BBC World Service to talk about back pain. We chatted about this problem of sitting too much and the interviewer made the point that in "hot countries" like India and Burma etc they generally sat on much more light weight chairs and settees etc because of the heat. In other words it would quickly become very uncomfortable to sit on the heavy, padded furniture that we are used to.

They squat as children right through to old age. Squatting is excellent because it is what the human body is designed to do. It moves the hips, knees and ankles through full range and it opens up the joints of the pelvis to self-correct any stiffening, or jamming of the joints at the bottom of the spine.

Children in the west also squat naturally, but lose the ability as they grow up and have to sit on chairs.

Of course the other issue is that the more sedentary we become in our relatively well-off Western society, then the heavier we become.

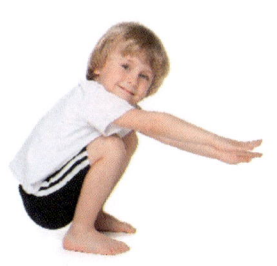

I will leave the discussion about diet, as we all know that we eat too much and the whole subject is best covered elsewhere by more competent people than me. But the additional weight loads all the joints of the back, hips, knees and feet.

I well remember reading somewhere that there is apparently a ton more Americans on the planet each day - not from population increase, but by *existing* people putting on weight. The UK cannot be far behind!

Obesity does not just mean the increased likelihood of diabetes, heart disease, stroke and cancer.

The problem as I see it, is not just the lack of exercise, too much food and excessive sitting. There is the other side of the problem in our modern healthcare system. **We have not recognised the problem as it was developing.**

We now have an epidemic of back pain to the extent that it has become part of our culture to actually expect to have low back pain at some point in our lives.

We all *expect* to end up with arthritis, walking frames and disability because there is this attitude from the healthcare professions that nothing can be done except a few painkillers and anti-inflammatories.

Basically, what do we expect – suck it up and live with it! Why should we?

I hope that by the time you have finished this book, you will be armed with all the information you need to prove the doctors wrong and to reduce the income to the drug companies!

I will feel that I may have done a good job if it gives you quality of life to be able to do all those things on your "bucket list" that you wouldn't otherwise have dared to attempt!

These short, but common scenarios are to give you an idea of what could be a progression along the "low back pain road":

EPISODE ONE - LOW BACK PAIN

The pain is relatively mild and the main pain is aching at the bottom of the back. It does not stop any particular movement, but it makes life a bit difficult.

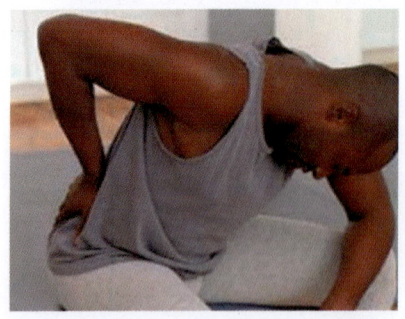

Friends and relatives say not to worry too much about it as you can still walk around; some people say you should go to bed for a couple of days; others say you should see your doctor and others recommend a local masseuse.

What you do is to take a few painkillers – Paracetamol, sit with a wheat bag (heated in a microwave) on your back when you get the opportunity and generally keep moving around to stretch the back as you find this the most useful thing to do.

At this level, you feel it is not worth bothering the GP about, so you are happy to try and manage this yourself.

After a couple of days, the aching has all but gone and you feel more confident to do more. You know that everything is moving in the right direction.

You still don't know what caused the low back pain, but you bow to popular opinion that it must have been a "strained muscle". You go back to work and think no more about it as after these few days, the pain has gone.

In this scenario, this is the first episode of low back pain that could be happening at almost any age.

It may have started after doing some digging in the garden, or starting some new sport. Or simply being under stress for some reason, not moving so easily, or having to do extra physical work. This maybe looking after a sick relative, or having to take on more at work.

Simple, short term pain relief such as Paracetamol.
Heat instead of cold. Wheatbags are easier to manage than hot water bottles.
Keep moving. Simple exercises. But keeping the head up every time bending forward.
Better within a few days
Back at work within the week.

COMMENT:

A detailed examination at this point from a specialist in MSK problems would have highlighted exactly what the problem was and how to avoid further episodes.

Unfortunately, fast referrals to NHS physiotherapy MSK specialists is seldom available, but this service is offered within the private sector – within 48 hours.

It is a great pity that this service is no longer on offer from the NHS as it is definitely the cost effective option to both you the patient and the NHS.

If you go to see the GP they will almost certainly think you have a "muscle strain" and prescribe NSAIDs and analgaesics.

Although you may be "better" within 6 weeks, you have lost that time from work.

EPISODE TWO - RECURRENCE OF LOW BACK PAIN

About three months down the line since the first episode, you slip over at work and fall on your bottom. You pick yourself up and think no more about it.

But a week later you bend over to pick up your shoe off the floor and suddenly you get a really sharp pain in the back. You manage to get to a chair and sit down, but the pain just gets worse. It starts to move into your right buttock.

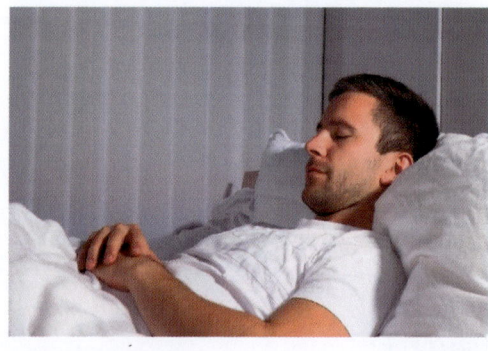

You take some Paracetamol and manage to get yourself home. You go to bed with a wheat bag.

Next day, your back is feeling a little easier and you try and get up and move around. You get an emergency appointment with your GP for the next day and you manage to get someone to take you to the surgery.

As this is the first time you have been to your GP for low back pain, and there are no obviously serious indicators such as incontinence, then he prescribes analgaesics and non-steroidal anti-inflammatories (NSAIDs) for an apparently more severe muscle strain in the low back.

Although the examination only took a few minutes, you appreciate that the GP is pushed for time, but he seemed confident in his assessment. So you take the prescription and go home.

The combination of painkillers and NSAIDs seems to be working and you mange to keep moving, although you can't go back to work yet.

Your GP tells you that most back pain will clear up within 6 weeks.

It takes a full six weeks before you are fit enough to go back to work and again this is time lost from work and normal activities.

THIRD EPISODE OF LOW BACK PAIN
far more severe and may include pain down the leg.

All seems well for the next year, but you wake up one morning with pain in the low back. As you get up, the pain goes down the leg and is now the worst pain. The pain in the low back seems to be getting less.

You can't get an appointment with the GP that day, so you try Paracetamol and Nurofen from the chemist. You use the wheat bag as before and try to keep moving, but the pain in the leg is still getting worse.

You see the GP the next day and he prescribes stronger analgaesics and NSAIDs.

You go back one week later as the pain is getting even more intense and you are finding the pain is stopping you sleeping. The GP refers you to the NHS Physiotherapy department, but the waiting list is about 2 months.

You go back to the GP 2 weeks later for stronger medication. The GP tries to get an urgent appointment with the Physiotherapists, but they still can't see you quickly.

Over the next week, the pain gets even worse and you find you are starting to lose the power of some of the muscles in the leg. You go back to the GP who refers you to the hospital to see an Orthopaedic Surgeon and arranges for an MRI in the meantime.

Two weeks later you have the MRI, but have to wait another 2 weeks for the results. It shows a large disc lesion at L5 S1, which is pressing on part of the sciatic nerve and causing the pain and muscle weakness in the leg. (This is the last disc in the spine between the 5th lumbar vertebra and the sacrum, which is the big triangular bone sitting in the pelvis. See Chapter 3 for the anatomy).

The appointment with the Orthopaedic Surgeon comes through, after another 2 weeks, by which time you have noticed that the leg from the knee down is numb as well as weak.

The Orthopaedic Surgeon decides that surgery is the best option and you agree. The surgery is carried out 2 weeks later – 3 months after the start of this episode. You have a short course of rehabilitation at an NHS Physiotherapy department, but there is still some pain and weakness in the leg, but not as severe as before the operation.

You were unable to go back to work before the surgery, but now have to stop work altogether even with the lower level of pain. You have to start claiming any allowances and benefits you can to pay your mortgage etc.

The pain remains at that level for the next 6 months and eventually the GP refers you to the Pain Clinic. They try different medication to start with and this slightly improves the pain, especially at night.

Over the next year, they try different approaches including injections and Cognitive Behavioural Therapy (CBT) as the problem is now very much a Chronic Pain condition. All of this input manages to reduce the pain to a manageable level, but you now have no possibility of returning to work. You have become part of the 7% that that take up 90% of the costs of low back pain.

Very typically, you then spend years going from one person to another trying to find an answer to the pain, including further surgery.

This very sorry state of affairs is not common, but it can and does happen.

Early intervention by a specialist MSK practitioner can stop this situation developing to this extent.

If this patient could have been seen early on by specialist MSK physiotherapists in the NHS, instead of the GP, or even the Orthopaedic Surgeon, then conservative treatment could have been given and the likelihood of being able to return to work would have been a definite possibility.

To have to wait so long with only increasing medication levels is really not acceptable. The cost of the medication and ultimately the surgery with all the people involved is considerably more than the cost of early conservative intervention.

Again, this is a service that is being picked up by the private sector. My advice is don't wait for the NHS.

Of course these are just hypothetical examples, but I hope you can see my point. get your back sorted out early, by an MSK specialist and you will save yourself (and the country!) a great deal of money, pain and stress.

Let's look at these scenarios in a little more detail

"Most low back pain is caused by straining a muscle" is a very common mis-diagnosis.

There are seven layers of back muscles. They vary in size from the small ones passing between the vertebrae, to the huge strap like muscles that cover almost the whole of the back. So which muscle, or part of a muscle was it that became "strained" or "pulled" to the exclusion of all the others?

Think about this for a moment. How do you damage a muscle?

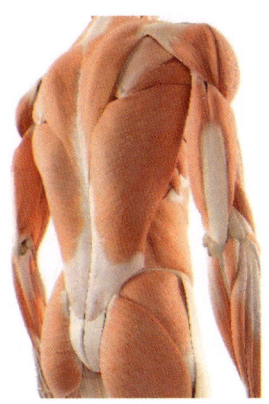

The most common way is to play sport where the muscles are put under tension and load which results in some or all of the fibres of the muscle being literally torn. If you tear just a few fibres, that this is classified as a grade 1. If you tear about half the thickness of the muscle then this would be a grade 2, and a complete thickness tear i.e. a complete rupture, is classified as a grade 3.

All three grades of damage will result in bleeding to a greater or lesser extent i.e. bruising. Depending on where the muscle is in your body, you may or may not actually see the bruising. The other important factor here is that muscles will take, on average, six weeks to heal if you do nothing to speed the process. I would suggest that this is why six weeks seems to be the golden timeframe applied to almost any musculoskeletal condition.

So there needs to be an injury. If there was an injury you would think that people would remember this as a specific incident, and yet a high proportion of people will come into the clinic with no memory of any injury or incident. Apart from direct trauma to the back i.e. a kick or a fall, I have yet to see any bruising associated with low back pain.

The other interesting fact is that by manipulating the joints in the back of someone with acute back pain, it is possible to restore all the movement and relieve the pain within a few moments. This either suggests that it is possible to cure muscle damage in a matter of moments using manipulation, or more likely, that in fact the problem was coming from joints.

It should be noted here, that manipulation is the technical term for a high velocity thrust technique designed specifically to restore movement to joints. It is a common misunderstanding that manipulation means almost any hands on technique, including massage and mobilisations, that are used to gently restore the movement of joints.

The fact that ligaments will take eight weeks to get better doesn't seem to figure in the equation! But then I guess any other soft tissue injury is included by making the patients wait for physiotherapy, or a consultant surgeon appointment.

Perhaps this is the secret! If you make the patients wait long enough for treatment, then they will get better without any further cost to the healthcare system! But what about the pain and suffering that has to be endured during that magic six or eight week window?

The spine has six layers of muscles and they all work to move the spine and to hold it in the right position. They allow us to move our arms and legs to perform a function like walking, or simply standing to use our arms to work etc. It would simply require a great deal of force to the muscles in the back and the likelihood of tearing just one of these muscles is extremely unlikely given that they work as a unit.

In other words, the simple act of bending over to pick your shoes off the floor requires a huge amount of muscle activity in the whole body and to tear just one of these is simply not possible. This is not opinion it is fact. There is no evidence to support this common "diagnosis".

I can accept that there may well be problems with the muscle system working to support, stabilise and move the spine, but these problems generally come on after an injury or problem to the joints. This is because any changes in the way that joints work will affect the way the muscles can work to move them.

These changes in the way that the muscles work can be classified in two ways:

Muscles on either side of the spine will tighten down to try and splint the damaged joints underneath. This is commonly known as "muscle spasm".

It is a protective mechanism designed to try and stop you damaging the joint even more. It is not exclusive to the spine. It will happen around virtually all joints that are damaged in some way.

The problem really starts when these muscles don't stop this splinting action. In effect what happens is that these muscles "screw" the joints down even tighter. This means that there is even more loss of movement in the joints below and it may well cause problems with surrounding joints in the spine that weren't affected by the original damage process. This is what people talk about when they say that their back has gone into "spasm". It is also why doctors may prescribe muscle relaxants, like diazepam, to try and stop this over-tightening effect of the muscles. The other issue here is that in itself, this muscle spasm is not painful.

The muscles themselves are not producing the pain.

You have a spinal joint that has suffered some damage.

This might be *direct* damage to some part of the joint, or

progressive loading causing wearing on that part of the joint. What then happens is that the muscles that should normally produce movement in the joint cannot work because the joint doesn't move in that way anymore. The muscles concerned then start to weaken and this has the knock-on effect of reducing the action of even more muscles that are designed to work alongside them.

For example, you want to reach forward to pick up a cup of tea off the table in front of you. This action requires you to bend forward slightly from the waist and reach forward with one arm.

Simple you think! But what is needed is for a whole group of muscles all over the body to work together as a unit at the right moment, to adjust the position of the body and to support all the joints involved in reaching your arm forwards for that cup of tea. If there is a fault in the line i.e. problems with part of the spinal joints needed to bend forward, then the muscles that should be making that movement can't carry out the action. The other muscles in the line then can't carry out their part either.

The body is very clever at overcoming this problem by moving other joints so that you can pick up a cup of tea. In other words, there are more ways than one to achieve the action. This change from the "normal" action means that some muscles will lose their part in making the movement happen.

If this goes on for a long time, then the body will make lasting changes to the way you move. You can see this very clearly in the different ways people walk. Someone with hip arthritis will walk very differently from someone with fully functioning hips.

As physiotherapists, we learn about all the structures that make up the human body. We learn about the joints, muscles and other soft tissues and how they work; the movements they can produce; how the body can perform all the movements that make us human. We learn what are the normal patterns of movement. We learn how to use this knowledge and understanding to re-educate movement patterns as well as any disease, dysfunction, injury and pain that may make the body move in abnormal ways.

What needs to be understood, *and remembered,* is that we learn patterns of movements depending on our joints. Though the basic structure of joints is pretty much the same, there will be differences in movement because of the differences in size, physical abilities, inherited flexibility. There are soft tissues and a whole host of other differences that go to make everyone of us unique individuals.

It is this complete individuality that should be appreciated and we need to consider when diagnosing the problem, the treatment techniques, the recovery and rehabilitation programs.

What can also make a huge difference to the way we move is our state of mind. It seems such an obvious thing to say. If we are feeling depressed or under the weather, then we move in very different ways from when we are on top of everything and the sun is shining! Very simply, posture changes. These changes will alter the loading through the joints and eventually lead to excessive wear with all the associated changes in the muscle groups that create the movement.

Over my 41 years as a physiotherapist there have been major advances in our understanding of how the muscle systems work to allow us to achieve the movements and actions that we need to function as people. These advances in our knowledge are the result of amazing research carried out by physiotherapists across the world. Physiotherapists such as the Australian Professor Paul Hodges, have been at the forefront of this work. (He has two PhD's – one in physiotherapy and the other in neuroscience!)

To get back to the three scenarios

GPs have on average 10 minutes to listen and understand the problems, the history, the symptoms and pain the patient is experiencing and then to examine him, decide on a possible diagnosis and suggest a possible course of action to try and resolve the problem.

This timescale is unrealistic and open to mistakes and errors. Yet this is what the average GP is expected to do in the NHS today. What I find remarkable is that all mistakes, errors and omissions are not more commonplace with all the resulting complaints litigation that can follow. The reality is that few people with musculoskeletal problems actually come to any serious harm if no treatment is offered at all!

We know that if people stopped going to their GP with low back pain then 90% would get better anyway!

All they need is simple pain control and advice about how to manage the problem. (Hence this book!) If they did, then the GP would be free to see those patients with potentially serious diseases etc and they would have far more time to spend at each consultation. This would allow them to do the job they were trained to do far more effectively, and cost effectively, to everyone's satisfaction.

Significant studies have been carried out that prove this is true and Health Authorities are very keen to give people with back pain a leaflet - as this is considerably cheaper than anything else! Fair comment you might think, but what about trying to stop the progression from simple low back pain through to major surgery, chronic pain and the enormous costs?

Unfortunately, this time constraint is not limited to GPs. Physiotherapists in the NHS are also being limited to 20 minutes. This is still not enough time to do the job properly and effectively. The other problem is the NHS waiting lists to see a physiotherapist in the first place! You could wait as much as six months or more for an NHS appointment and then you get just 20 minutes, which is hardly worth having. Perhaps the same argument applies?

Doctors and physiotherapists can complain all they like about these time constraints, as patients don't generally die of MSK problems, so they are not seen as a priority for NHS spending. As with so much these days, it all comes back to money! Not the patient's money of course, the NHS budget. This patient could've been a self-employed builder with the family and mortgage to support. Not being able to work for six weeks because of his back pain could well have put him at risk of losing contracts, his work, his house and even his family.

I'm not saying that money should be diverted from excellent emergency services; the heart unit; cancer treatment and all the other incredibly important lifesaving areas of work. It is just that there needs to be a change in the way the NHS looks at MSK problems in light of the effect that poor service and treatment has on the individuals, as well as the overall economy of the country.

Accident and emergency departments should have MSK physiotherapy specialists to deal with all the sprained ankles and bad backs in minor injuries. This would leave the doctors free to deal with the medical emergencies. These specialist physiotherapists would certainly have the knowledge to know if the patient has something more serious and they would be in the ideal place to pass the patient quickly to the doctors in A and E for medical assessment and investigations if necessary.

This idea has recently been recommended by the CEO of the Chartered Society of Physiotherapy (CSP), as a sensible and cost-effective way of dealing with increasing attendance rate of patients to A and E.

The problem appears to me to be the reluctance of the medical profession to relinquish part of the A and E departments to physiotherapists, as well as a lack of understanding of the skills and specialist knowledge of physiotherapists, by the politicians and NHS managers.

I do hope that a politician is reading this book, as the CSP press release was largely ignored by the media - and government! (January 2015)

Back pain costs the NHS of the country more than any other single condition – £3 billion a year to the UK economy!

If the service provided was effective and efficient then there would be huge savings to be made to the country, to the GP budgets, industry and most importantly to the individual patients and their lives. To provide a service that is expensive at best, yet ineffective, is financial lunacy! I moved out of the NHS 35 years ago, because I realised that it was impossible to provide efficient and cost-effective treatment for MSK problems in the hospital setting.

In the private sector it is possible to offer the most effective service, and if this didn't work then I would've been out of business years ago. And yet the NHS still thinks the answer is to throw money at the problem without understanding the right treatment by the right professionals is the most cost-effective route for all.

Doctors should not be the first port of call for patients with MSK problems. This absolutely should be a specialist MSK physiotherapist. Studies and pilot projects have shown this approach works, but **still** there is this idea that physiotherapists who have specialised in MSK problems do not have the knowledge to be able to provide the service. Most doctors have no idea of the level of knowledge, training and skill of physiotherapists because, as a profession, we have not told them! Very few doctors have even set foot inside the physiotherapy department.

After 120 years, physiotherapy is only really appreciated by physiotherapists! I still get patients who are amazed that physiotherapy is a degree course at university. The image is still one of heat, massage and exercises that only need a few weekend courses to achieve.

In reality the BSc courses are made up of 4000 hours and have to include at least 1000 hours of clinical placement for physiotherapists to be eligible for membership of the Chartered Society of Physiotherapy (CSP). The CSP is our professional body.

Equally, there is the misconception that all physiotherapists are the same and that there is no further learning needed once you have the degree. In other words there is little general understanding that there actually is a career progression dependent on the postgraduate training.

We all have to undertake postgraduate courses to maintain our membership of the Chartered Society of Physiotherapy and to be registered members of the Health Care Professions Council, which is a legal requirement that allows us to treat patients. Most of us keep learning throughout our postgraduate lives and enjoy the process of keeping up-to-date with the latest research, as well as learning new treatment and diagnostic techniques.

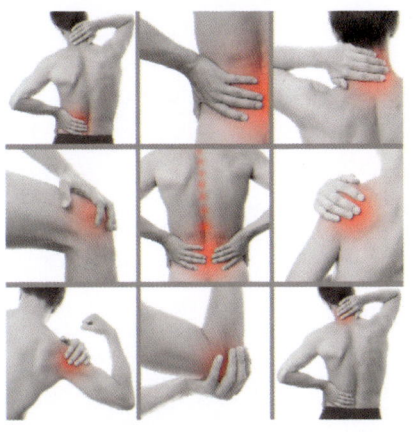 The pity is the salaries are not directly linked to postgraduate training and there are physiotherapists working in the NHS who have PhDs, but were being put onto salary scales, under the NHS Agenda for Change, alongside staff who only have the basic BSc degrees. All of this is down to our profession and will only change when we learn to promote the benefits of our work - for the patient, the NHS and society at large.

Chapter 3

THE BACK EXAMINATION

As a starting point to help you get the best advice and treatment for your low back pain, I am going to give you the information to find out whether you are actually getting the best advice.

There are so many people out there who claim to be able to "cure" back pain, or at least manage it, and yet they have virtually no knowledge, experience or qualifications to support their claims. This doesn't help *you*, the patient, in trying to find someone who can help.

There are endless numbers of people who will offer you advice based on their own experiences, or what they have read in a newspaper or magazine. Please beware of this sort of advice.

Your experience is different from everyone else. How *you* respond to a painful condition is different and is going to be based on all *your* past experiences; *you* as a person; the impact of this condition on *your* life and *your* expectations and fears.

It is all of these considerations that have to be taken into account when we, as Health Professionals who are trained and experienced in this field, decide on the best treatment options for *you* as an individual. What works for some people, does not work for others for many and varied reasons.

Only 40% of people with low back pain go to their GP

Understandably it seems, most people will go to someone who is recommended to them by friends or family purely on results.

That is not too much of a problem until you look a little deeper. What if something goes wrong with your treatment? Does this person have Professional Indemnity insurance because of their recognised qualifications? Do they have any recognised and validated qualifications at all? Where do you go to find out? Equally, how much post graduate knowledge and experience does this healthcare practitioner have? Who actually does have the required undergraduate qualification?

It is an absolute minefield!

Do you need:

- A physiotherapist?
- Your GP?
- An orthopaedic surgeon?
- A rheumatologist?
- An osteopath?
- A chiropractor?
- A sports therapist?
- The pharmacist at the local chemist?
- A massage?

You need sound, reasoned advice, and that is what I am hoping to give you here. If you know what is wrong, or at least have a good idea what is going on, then you will have a fighting chance of seeing the right person at the right time. (You will have realised that I will always put physiotherapist at the top of the list - if they have the right post graduate, specialist knowledge and training!)

To try and make this easier to follow, I have written this where "you" means the patient and "we", or "I", means the examining healthcare professional who might be a physiotherapist, doctor, osteopath or chiropractor as these are the most appropriate professionals who see patients with musculoskeletal conditions including low back pain.

It is divided into two main sections and is the same for any musculoskeletal condition.

1. The **subjective** examination is where all the information is collected about the problem. This should include the immediate history of the problem and anything that could be related, family

history, work, injuries, other medical conditions, any traffic accidents or falls, slips and slides.

All of this comes from asking you for the details and from any medical records that we may already have on file if you've been seen before.

At the end of the subjective examination, there should be a clear timeline of all the events that have led up to your asking for help and treatment on that day.

2. The **objective** examination is where all the clinical tests are carried out to objectively test any ideas/hypotheses/possible diagnoses and possible causes of the pain and problems identified in the subjective examination.

The objective examination is split into sections which test the different structures that could be causing the problem.

Passive movements. These test the **joints** and look at the available range of movement that can be limited (compare to the so-called normal or expected ranges).

Active movements. These test the range of movement that *you*, the patient, can move the joints. Limitation in the active ranges can be either from changes within the joints, weakness of the muscles that move the joints, compression on the nerves, or pain.

Resisted movements. (Or myotomes) These test the strength of the associated muscle groups, which could be limited/weak because of injury to the muscles, which will cause pain when the muscle contracts, or there is a problem with the nerve supply to the muscles. Weakness can also be caused through disuse, where the muscles have not been able to work because of restricted joint movement.

Neural tests. These are used to test the *conductivity* of the nerves in question. For patients with low back pain, this will include the ankle and knee jerks and a test called the Babinski, or plantar response. This last one involves "scraping" the end of the reflex hammer up the sole of the foot. If the test is positive, then there may be a chance of more serious pathology and needs a Consultant referral.

Neurodynamic tests. These test the ability of the nerves to move and stretch. If they are stuck somewhere then there will be a painful response to the test as well as limited range of movement. They include the Straight Leg Raise (SLR) for the sciatic nerve in particular, but also include looking at the mobility of the spinal cord itself.

Skin tests. If the previous tests suggest that the nerves are being compressed, then there is the possibility that the sensory nerves in the skin could be affected leading to reduction or loss of sensation ie partial or total numbness in specific areas of the skin supplied by the nerve in question.

Loss of skin sensation, with or without muscle weakness, in an area that is *not* supplied by the nerves in question, could indicate a more serious problem and need a Consultant referral.

At the end of this section, there should be clear evidence of the injury or condition, which will then lead to a treatment programme designed to sort out the problem. If no clear diagnosis comes out of the objective examination then it may be necessary to refer you for a more detailed examination that would include x-rays, scans and/or blood tests etc. There are also special tests that are used to indicate any serious pathology, which if found, will obviously mean a referral to the appropriate consultant.

You can see from this that when these examinations are carried out with all the required detail and precision, it becomes a very valuable tool in the diagnosis and treatment of MSK conditions. The problem with most MSK conditions is that we cannot actually see them, and we cannot find them with specific blood tests.

Precisely identifying the structure that is causing the pain takes great skill, knowledge and expertise.

What must not be forgotten in all this information is your attitudes and beliefs. This can have a definite impact on the results of various tests and needs to be taken into account.

For example, you may have a great fear that something very serious is causing the problem and you may subconsciously "tighten up" when the tests are being carried out. The increased tension in various muscle groups can reduce ranges of movement in joints that an inexperienced healthcare professional may not be able to identify. He would then assume that there is a greater loss of range of movement than there actually is. This in turn could lead to wrong assumptions and therefore a wrong diagnosis.

With a wrong diagnosis, the wrong treatment could be offered, which at worst could be harmful and at best would be ineffective.

The other problem with these sorts of conditions is that doctors in particular tend to rely heavily on what can be seen, measured and recorded with *medical* tests such as scans and blood tests and this can lead to treatments that are completely wrong in particular circumstances.

Of course, there is nothing wrong with the medical approach, and it works very well for the diagnosis of diseases and trauma. In these circumstances there are tangible changes within the body that actually *can* be seen and measured. It would be really good if this also applied to musculoskeletal conditions, but it doesn't!

We may be able to see the damage to a ligament in the ankle with an MRI, but it won't tell us how much pain you are experiencing, or even whether the pain is actually coming from that structure at all. It may be referred to the ankle from an injury to the low back when you fell over and sprained the ankle. It might be 6 of one and half a dozen of the other.

No scan can tell us that and even the scanning system in Star Trek is not going to be able to tell us, because we are dealing with individual people!

This short case study will show you what I mean:

A previous patient of mine, in her 70s, came into the clinic complaining of a mild low back pain. We carried out the clinical examination and decided that the cause of the pain was a small joint problem in the sacro-iliac joints. This was a very simple problem for us, which settled well with a low grade manipulation and Interferential Therapy (a type of electrotherapy designed to increase the blood supply and healing rate, which I have been working with since 1978).

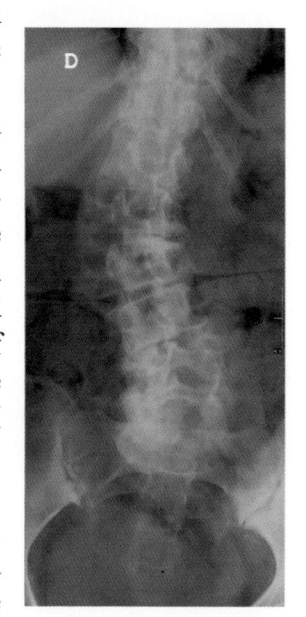

She then went away on holiday, but some of the back pain returned (maybe as a result of sitting on the plane for a time) within a couple of days of having the treatment.

She went along to see a local doctor while she was on holiday and he thought it might be an idea for her to have an MRI of her back, just to see what might be going on there. When the results came back, he was horrified to see that the bones and joints at the bottom of the spine were misshapen and even twisted.

His advice to her was that she should see a Neurosurgeon as soon as she got home. Instead, she came to see me again to ask if she should see a consultant. We examined her again and still there were very few signs and symptoms and she still only had a mild, but irritating pain in her low back. All the special tests we carried out showed no problems and no reason for her to see a consultant. We treated her as before and the pain went away.

This proved to be a classic situation where what was seen on the scan did not match the clinical signs and symptoms. In fact, with her permission, I have a copy of the X ray to demonstrate the point to the physiotherapy students that we have on clinical placement from the universities. The changes in the bone and joint alignment must have taken many years to develop and the body has an incredible capacity for sorting out problems on its own!

In this case what had happened was that the body had laid down bone to deal with the changes in the loading through the joints. It effectively *strutted* that part of the spine so it couldn't't move anymore. (This is what the surgeons would do if there was a risk of the vertebrae moving enough to put the spinal cord at risk). It wasn't something new. It would have taken more than 20 years to slowly change like that.

If this patient had gone to see a Consultant, then he may very well have recommended surgery to try and make the spine "normal". But this would have taken away the stable structure that the body had worked so hard to achieve in favour of something that looked like the pictures in Gray's Anatomy! The surgery itself could well have caused far more pain than the original condition.

Exactly this scenario happened with another patient of mine who was busy walking up and down mountains, but was getting a relatively small amount of back pain with occasional pain into the leg. The consultant looked at the scans and X rays and saw a grossly distorted lumbar spine. He then operated and put in two big rods to straighten and fix the spine.

This patient then suffered enormously from the surgery and even developed problems with his heart and lungs as a direct result of the massive amount of medication that he had to take. The irony is that after more than a year following the surgery, he still had the original pain. This proved that the abnormal position of the spine was not the cause of his problems!

Just to make the point again, what is seen on X rays or scans isn't necessarily the cause of the problem or the pain.

Now let's look at these elements of the examination in more detail:

THE SUBJECTIVE EXAMINATION

The Subjective Examination is a detailed question and answer session that allows you to present all the history/timeline/signs and symptoms of the reason why you are now sitting in front of me. There are key questions that should be asked of you to help identify any possible serious condition that would require referring you to say, an orthopaedic surgeon.

These *special* questions should include asking whether you have any problems with your bladder and bowel.

This is because there could be a problem if you are losing control of passing water. In other words you are losing *control* of the sphincters of the bladder and bowel. If this is happening, then there may be a part of the disc between the spinal vertebrae pressing so hard on the spinal cord that the nerves to the sphincters are not working. This is a serious situation and means that the disc material should be removed surgically within 48 hours. Otherwise, the nerves could be damaged and the incontinence could be permanent.

Another *special* situation could be where there is pain down *both* legs as this could mean that both sciatic nerves are being compressed at the same time. There are very few situations where this can happen, but one of them could be where the disc "bulge" is so great that it has spread out to squeeze the nerves on either side of the spine.

It is not uncommon to get pain down just one leg from disc material pressing on a branch of the sciatic nerve; or where the sacro-iliac joint on one side is putting a stretch on the nerve; or where the facet joint on one side has closed down on the emerging nerve. A relatively mild compression of the nerve will cause pain, but if this compression increases then you may start to lose muscle power and sensation in that part of the leg that the nerve supplies.

If you put even more load on the nerve, then the reflexes can be affected. If you get pain, muscle weakness *and* loss of sensation in the leg, then again this needs surgery. In extreme cases all the pain disappears, you lose the strength in your leg, or you can't pull your foot up towards you, or stand on tiptoe on that side, *and* you cannot feel anything when parts of your leg are touched, then again surgery is needed as soon as it can be arranged otherwise there may be permanent damage to the nerve.

Remember though, these situations are rare. If there is any doubt then this would be a situation for the doctors and not physiotherapists, osteopaths or chiropractors, or sports masseur, or anyone else. So get an urgent appointment with your GP and don't take "No" from the GP receptionists!

In general terms, at the end of this discussion we should have a very clear understanding of what has happened to you as well as the progress of the condition since it first started. With low back pain in particular, a good 80% of the diagnosis can be made from this discussion. It will be almost a 100% certainty that your problem is not down to a muscle injury in the back

THE OBJECTIVE EXAMINATION OR PHYSICAL EXAMINATION

For this you should be asked to undress down to your underwear. It is only by looking at the whole body in standing, sitting or lying that you can see where the problems might lie. Equally, it is not possible to test the reflexes, or test for loss of skin sensation or muscle power through trousers!

To break this part of the examination into some sort of logical progression means that you can begin to understand what is being done and why!

Observation

Before actually looking at how the spine moves, it is vitally important to see how you are generally moving and to see how you hold your body in response to any problem when standing.

A very good example of this is the patient who comes in with a definite spinal shift to one side. They seem to be standing and moving, but with the spine shifted off to one side.

Technically, this can be described as a "scoliosis", which means that the spine has taken up a position that off loads the problem area. 9 times out of 10 this is a specific indicator of an L4 disc lesion and we can make this diagnosis simply by watching the way the patient walks across the car park! This phenomenon happens because of a quirk in the anatomy configuration at that level.

Just looking at someone from behind, provides us with a significant number of pointers for certain diagnoses. It will be necessary to have you undressed to the underwear as we cannot see these differences and indicators through clothes!

As physiotherapists, we are trained to look, and to *see*, these indicators:

1. Symmetry in the trunk
2. The way the head is held in relation to the neck and shoulders
3. Are the lower angles of the shoulder blades level?
4. Are the curves at the waist the same on each side?
5. Is the chest and trunk rotated on the pelvis?
6. Is the pelvis rotated on its horizontal axis?
7. Is it rotated on its vertical axis?
8. Are the buttock creases level?
9. Are the knee creases level?
10. Are there problems with the feet?

These are the main things we are looking at, but there are many more. We are looking for signs that fit with the history.

JOINTS THAT MAY BE AT FAULT

What we are looking for here is to find out which joints, if any, are the source of the problem. There are particular areas that we want to know about:

Pain (remembering that these examinations are trying to find the cause of the pain). What movements cause a change in the pain? This maybe an increase or a decrease.

Mechanical blockage, such as "slipped disc" or arthritis. What movements are limited compared to others?

Increased tension in the surrounding muscles trying to protect the joint underneath. Is there an increase in muscle tone and which muscles are working to perform the movement?

(please note: the pain is *not* coming from the muscles themselves. This protective tension causes a tightening down of the joints underneath)

Diseases that affect the joints such as tumours, osteoporosis etc that need referral for a Consultant opinion. In other words, diseases and conditions that are not going to respond to conservative treatment.

THE PASSIVE MOVEMENTS OF THE LOW BACK

In order to see if there are problems with the joints, then we need to move them in a way that is called "Passive movements". To be able to do this we need to have a detailed knowledge of the range of movement that *should* be there in a so called "normal" individual. This then gives us a reference point to compare.

If we are looking at knees, for example, you generally have two knees and we can then compare the left with the right, but when we are dealing with the spine then there is only one spinal column! We also need to take into account your age and general fitness to decide what joint movement is normal for you and when something has gone a bit wrong!

As I have said before, you should be asked to undress down to your underwear in order that the movements you will be asked to perform can be seen.

There are 4 standard movements of the low back and these are performed in standing.

You are asked to bend backwards, sideways to the left and then to the right, (or right then left if you prefer!) and then to try and touch your toes.

These movements appear to be very simple, but what we have to remember is that the body moves to achieve a *function* and not an *action*. In other words, when the task "try and touch your toes" is given, the body does exactly that. It doesn't "consider" **how** it does it, only that it will bring into play every muscle etc. needed, at that moment, to **achieve** the task. What we will be looking for is any abnormal muscle and joint activity brought in to play when the task is carried out. This will give us a clear indication of possible problems.

It is amazing how the body will compensate and find another way of performing the task. The most obvious example is limping after spraining your ankle. Perhaps one of the least obvious to the untrained eye is the start of arthritis in the hip, or a tendon problem in the shoulder.

There has been a great deal of research into this adaption process and the Physiotherapy profession is at the forefront of this area of work, because our core knowledge is movement of the human body, and how to restore movement after injury, surgery or disease.

As a point of interest - asking you to bend backwards, forwards and sideways are apparently *active* movements ie **you** initiate the movement, but because of the effect of gravity these particular movements are in fact *passive* movements of the joints involved. You start the movement, but gravity then takes over for you.

There have been any number of examples of equipment that are designed to try and measure the individual movements of the joints in the low back. The problem is that even if it were possible to do this, then the essential compensatory movements would be missed. What the designers of these gizmos don't understand is that the body moves as a whole unit and any attempt to measure individual joint ranges actually misses the point. We need to be able to assess the whole body movement, action and function.

In fact the most useful assessment tool is a video camera and then slowing the film down to be able to analyse all the components that make up that whole movement. Analysis of what is actually going on relies on the knowledge and skill of the person looking at the video/patient.

It is really not possible to accurately quantify this aspect of the examination in terms of some measuring device that says the body has moved so many degrees this way and so many degrees that way, because all the reference markers are on the skin and skin moves. Not to put too fine a point on it, it is far easier to find the necessary surface markers and bony landmarks on someone who has very little body fat. Even then it can be difficult. You can mark the skin over a bony points with a felt tip pen, but as soon as you ask them to move, the skin will stretch and move as well. So the marked point will no longer be over that bony point. It is not an exact science!

The movement of the body is equally not that simple. There are too many variables and too many different ways that the body can perform tasks and actions. Every person will perform the action or task in a slightly different way depending on their age, health, muscle activity and strength, willingness to carry out the action, pain, and joint condition. This means that there are ranges of movement that fall within a normal range for that person, at that time in their lives. So the skill is deciding when this has become abnormal – for them! We once had a patient who had a spine tattooed over his spine! We had to do all the palpation with our eyes closed because the tattooist was not accurate with his in the placement of his tattoo!

This is what makes research difficult in the musculo-skeletal world!

HYPERMOBILITY

Before going on to the rest of the examination, I want to talk about **hypermobility.**

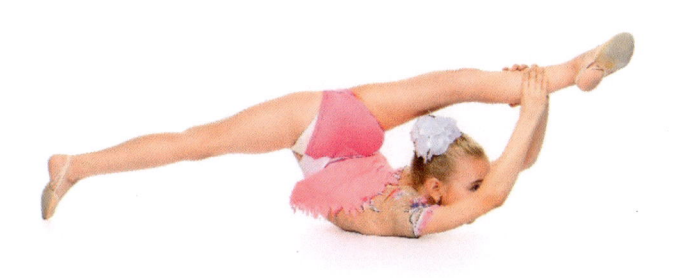

We inherit 80% of our flexibility from our parents. What we are specifically talking about here is the relative "length and stretch-ability" of the ligaments and connective tissues of the body. This is why some people can fold themselves up and fit themselves into a suitcase that would pass a budget airline requirement for luggage, and other people who, despite a huge amount of effort, have never been able to even touch their toes in standing!

One of my patients has managed to achieve a 4th Dan Black belt in Shotokan karate, but he still can't touch his toes! This is an excellent example of how the body can adapt its movement and function to suit its actual physical capability.

There are many grades of hypermobility and the standard assessment tool is the Beighton Scale to give a sort of "entry level" to the level of flexibility. It is thought that about 15 to 20% of the population have hypermobility that will fit into this scale.

At this lower level, it is not a major problem but still needs to be taken into account when assessing joint ranges and even more importantly when deciding what treatment systems and exercises are needed. However, what should also be taken into account is that there is an enormous variation from a degree of being "double jointed" to the other end of the scale with conditions such as Marfans or Ehlers-Danlos syndrome. These conditions at the far end of the scale involve the connective tissue of the *whole* body and include the tissues of the organs, which in turn leads to a wide variety of symptoms and problems over and above the increased flexibility, and resultant instability of the joints.

Marfans and Ehlers Danlos sufferers represent a very small percentage of people with hypermobility. So, let's look at the "average" person with a relatively low level of hypermobility. Their increased flexibility is often missed during an objective examination. Unless we are aware of the condition, then assumptions can be made about the available range of movement.

I like to explain this relative flexibility by thinking of dog breeds! What I mean by this is that some people are born Staffordshire terriers ie they are compact and strong, but with limited ranges of movement. These are the people who live in gyms, working hard to increase their strength and power. If they actually do any stretching at all they will struggle to gain any increase in the joint ranges. As I said, we inherit 80% of our flexibility, so we only have 20% to work on.

Then there are people who are born as the Afghan hounds of the human world! Having said that, our latest dog is an adolescent German Shepherd and he is also very flexible in that he can lie with his front paws folded under his wrists and with one paw behind his ear! He will often lie with his back legs and pelvis lying one way, but his front legs, trunk and head are facing the other.

Our Staffy cross, on the other hand, cannot put both front paws on the ground when she lies on her side!

Afghans in particular are slim and built for speed and flexibility. They are the track athletes of the dog world and their human equivalents are lithe, flexible and built for short bursts of speed. They will never be weight lifters, but they will be swimmers and gymnasts.

These differences in flexibility and body type are very important when carrying out a clinical examination of the musculo-skeletal system.

If they are not taken into account, then there is the very real possibility of making the wrong diagnosis.

BEIGHTON SCALE

The Beighton modification of the Carter & Wilkinson scoring system has been used for many years as an indicator of widespread hypermobility. A high Beighton score by itself does not mean that an individual has Hypermobility Syndrome (HMS). It simply means that the individual has widespread hypermobility.

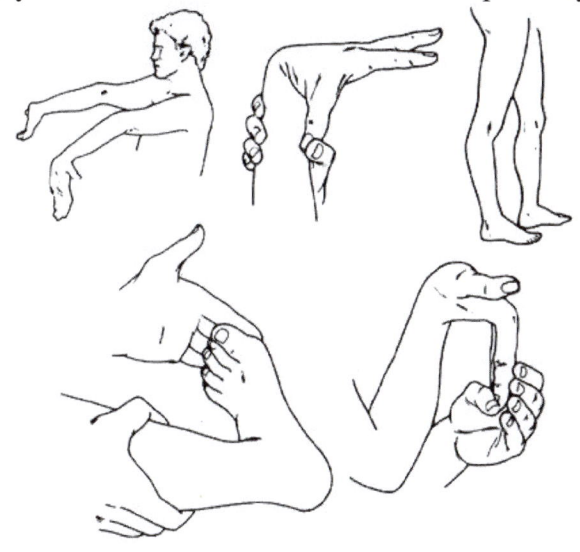

The Beighton score is calculated as follows:

Score one point if you can bend and place you hands flat on the floor without bending your knees.
Score one point for each elbow that will bend backwards (over straighten)
Score one point for each hand when you can bend the little finger back beyond 90°
Score one point for each knee that will bend backwards (over-straighten)

Score one point for each thumb that will bend down to touch the forearm

If you are able to perform all of above manoeuvres then you have a maximum score of 9 points.

Hypermobility simply means "excessive mobility". In other words your joints have an unusually wide range of movement. This is more than the average person's, which allows you to perform movements that are not available to most people.

It is what people often call "double jointed" or "very supple".

INFORMATION POINT: Ligaments can't contract like muscles. They act like "guy ropes" to stop the joints from moving beyond their normal range of movement and they are generally arranged around the joints where the greatest strain is applied. Tendons, on the other hand, attach muscles to the bones. When ligaments are "slacker" than average, as in people with Hypermobility, then there is far more "play" in ALL the joints.

For example, hypermobile people often find that they can write more easily with a fat pen. This means that they can control the movement of the fingers better than with a slim pen. This can cause children to become very frustrated as they go through to the senior school when they have to write more and they find they physically can't write quickly enough.

This laxity in the joints also mean that they need to work all the "stabiliser" muscles much more than the average person, in order to prevent possible damage to the joints.

Most people who are hypermobile do not realise that they are, but as they get older and start to stiffen up, they find it even more surprising to hear that they have this condition.

The majority of people with Hypermobility suffer no ill effects. In fact, they often excel in sports such as ballet and athletics where they use their hypermobility to advantage. If their joints are in good alignment and the muscles are toned up, then any symptoms are less likely to arise from hypermobility.

However, a small proportion of people with hypermobility do suffer from aching joints, especially after exercise, or aching legs. They find that standing for long periods gives them backache. They also tend to bruise more easily.

BACK TO THE EXAMINATION

As you are still standing at this point, it is a good time to test for any weakness in the calf muscles.

To do this, we ask you to stand on your toes, then to stand on the toes on one leg and then on the other. This is also a simple test for balance and will show any reluctance to perform this action that might be limited because of pain or something more complicated that might have gone wrong with the body's balance mechanisms.

These muscles in the calves are usually very strong as they work against gravity, to lift the body as we walk and move around, let alone running and jumping! They give us the spring in our walk and help to off load the forces going through the weight bearing joints such as the hips, knees and the spine. If they become weak, then we walk with a solid and plodding gait, because we have lost the bounce that the calves give us.

Unfortunately, this weakness can come on as we get older, as much because we stop running and jumping, as a factor of ageing. Very, very simply, muscles have either fast acting or slow acting fibres. The fast acting fibres are just that – they provide speed of action and are the main propulsive muscles that allow us to run and jump and generally to move at speed. The slow acting fibres equally do just that – they are the ones that help to keep us in the balanced position to be able to then use the fast acting fibred muscles to perform the tasks.

They are the postural muscles that allow us to use our arms and legs while providing a relatively solid body/structure as a support for the movement.

Weakness in one of the calf muscles could be as a result of the nerve that supplies them being squashed where it emerges from the spine. This is at the level of the disc between the 5th vertebra and the sacrum ie the last disc of the spine itself.

If both calf muscles are weak then this can be an indicator of more serious problems.

It is unlikely, but not impossible, for the disc material to involve both nerves as they come out of the spine on either side and cause the nerve compression and muscle weakness. This is a rare situation that can only really be dealt with by surgically removing the disc material.

There are a number of other causes of weakness in both legs, but these are generally neurological problems and not musculo-skeletal. There will be other signs and symptoms that will point to this as we go through the full examination to back up the thought that this needs a referral to the appropriate consultant for medical tests.

This ability to find out which nerve, or part of the nerve is involved, comes from knowing exactly what muscles, joints and skin are supplied by which nerve. Where there are signs and symptoms found in the different areas of the body, then it is possible to say where the problem tissue lies.

A good example of this is arthritis in the hip. The hip joint is supplied by the 3rd lumbar nerve, but there is also a feedback system from the skin down the front of the thigh, so pain from an arthritic hip is felt down the front of the thigh, the front of the knee and the front of the shin.

JOINTS OF THE HIP

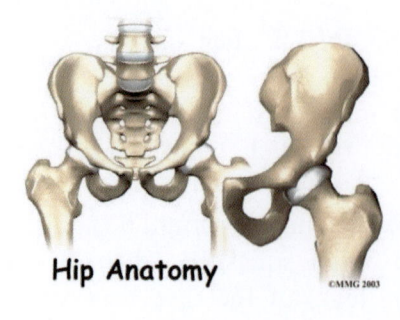

Hip Anatomy

This whole system of examination is designed to move you, the patient, as little as possible while respecting the fact that you may be in great pain and any movement is difficult. You don't want to be asked to stand up, sit down, lie down, turn over, stand up again etc as this may only make matters worse.

The next part of the examination needs you lying down on your back on the treatment couch.

In this position, we can move each hip in turn, working through all the available movements of the hip to see if they are limited in range, or cause pain.

The movements here are:

Flexion (bending the hip up to the chest)
Abduction (taking the leg out to the side)
Adduction (taking the leg across the body towards the other leg)
Internal or medial rotation (taking the hip and knee to about 90 degrees and then rotating the knee towards the other leg, and the foot out to the side)
External or lateral rotation (bending the hip and knee to 90 degrees again, but this time rotating the knee out to the side and the foot towards the other leg)

These movements tell us what range of movement is available in the hip joints, comparing one side with the other. Passive movements like these will tell us if the joint range is limited, but not necessarily what is causing the limitation.

There is a wonderful term we use and that is "end feel"! This is the sensation that we can pick up when actually moving the joint for you. There is a "hard end feel" which tells us that the joint has come up against a hard block. This is usually as a result of arthritis.

On this point of arthritis in joints, it is worth noting that the word "arthritis" actually means "inflammation in the joint". It doesn't't tell you what has caused the inflammation, or if it is a temporary problem or a long term one.

This needs other tests to make that decision, such as blood tests if the arthritis is being caused by a disease, or X rays and scans if it is caused by the wear and tear type osteoarthritis.

One very interesting fact is that all joints will become limited in a very specific way with osteoarthritis. This is because the capsule of the joint that holds all the insides of the joint in, becomes tight in certain areas when there is damage to the joint surfaces inside. We know that each joint has its own capsular pattern.

If we find that the hip is limited in the joint specific capsular pattern, then we know there is osteoarthritis present in that joint. The question then is, "How much is the arthritis contributing to the current problem?" Just because the joint is wearing out a bit, does not mean that it is the cause of the problem.

What this situation means is that there needs to be a full clinical examination to get to the real cause of the problem. Just because some abnormality is seen on X rays or scans, does not automatically mean that it must be causing the problem. The X ray/scan findings need to correlate with the clinical findings.

What is commonly missed is that if you move your hip up towards your chest (hip flexion) and you go beyond 90 degrees, then you are starting to rotate the pelvis bone. So if there is pain, or limitation at more than 90 degrees, then this could be the hip, but it is more than likely to be a sacroiliac joint issue.

The Straight Leg Raise (SLR).

The SLR belongs to a family of tests known as Neurological tests and as the name implies are designed to test the nerves. In this case, the sciatic nerve, specifically. We can gather a lot of information from this test when performed correctly. But let's have a quick look at the anatomy of this nerve first.

The sciatic nerve is the largest nerve in the body in all senses. It is both the longest and the thickest, as thick as your thumb, where it passes under the bony bit of your bottom. In other words, when you sit down, you are actually sitting on the sciatic nerve.

This fact would suggest that we are not designed to sit on chairs at all.

THE SCIATIC NERVE

(There is no exam for you at the end of this!)

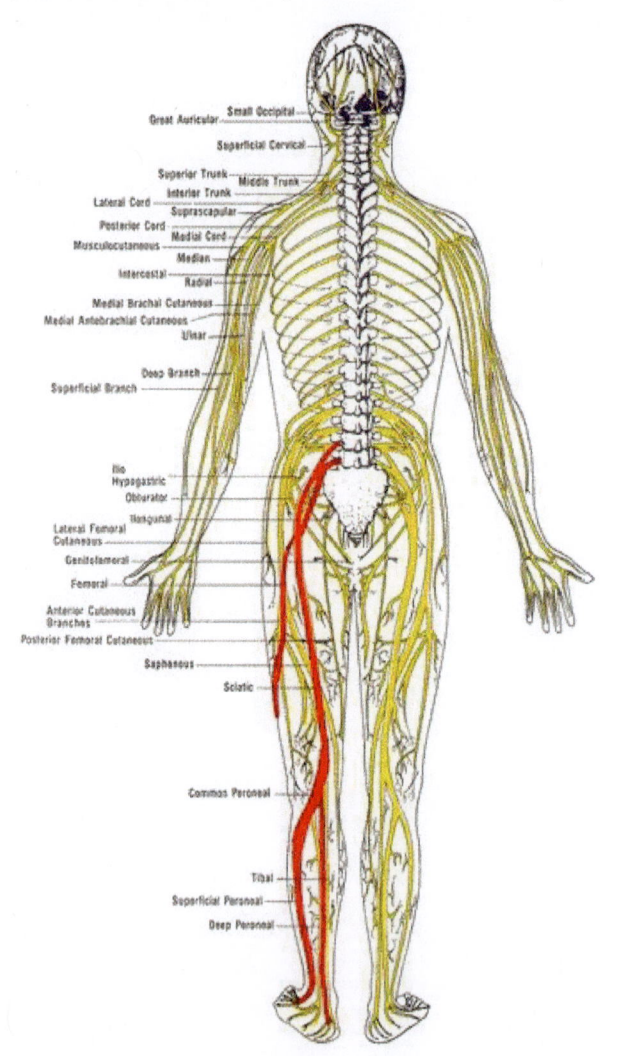

The sciatic nerve is made up of nerve roots that come out on either side of the last two lumbar vertebrae and out of the holes in the sacrum. All these roots join together to form the nerve. It passes through the pelvis and under the bony part of the bottom – technically known as the ischial tuberosity. From there it goes straight down through the back of the thigh to the back of the knee. Here it divides into two nerves, the common peroneal nerve and the tibial nerve.

The common peroneal nerve winds round the outside of the knee and down the outside of the calf. It then goes into the foot under the ankle bone medial malleolus) on the inside of the ankle and ends up on the big toe side of the top of the foot.

The tibial nerve on the other hand, goes down the middle of the back of the calf and goes into the foot around the ankle bone (lateral malleolus) on the outside of the foot.

There are a number of other nerves that come off the sciatic nerve and go into the leg at various points, but as this is not intended to be a full anatomy text, I am only going to talk about the common peroneal and the tibial nerves as they are the main ones to think about. If you want to know more then you can ask "Prof Google" or get a copy of Gray's Anatomy!

What I want to explain is that if you know your anatomy then you can put the respective nerves on the stretch. Then if a particular stretch is painful, then we know that the nerve is cross and upset somewhere along its length. The next thing to work out is where the problem lies along the length of the sciatic nerve.

The SLR is exactly that. You lie on your back on the treatment couch and we take hold of your leg and lift it for you – straight up until we hit the pain point, or the end of the range for that movement. We then hold the end position and pull your toes towards your head. This increases the stretch on the sciatic nerve and we need to know whether that increases the pain, or just increases the stretch in the leg.

The next add on is to keep the tension on and rotate the leg in so that your toes turn towards the other foot. This puts even more stretch on the sciatic nerve and its branches and yet again we need to know whether these staged increases in stretch and tension increase any pain, or simply an increased stretch throughout the leg? But this is not the end of the test! What we then ask you to do is to lift your head off the pillow, while we maintain the stretch on the leg and nerves.

The question asked now is, "Is the pain better, worse or the same when you lift your head off the pillow?"

Lifting your head off the pillow with a full SLR as described, puts the stretch on the spinal cord as well as the sciatic nerve and even includes a stretch on the meninges that surround the brain. In other words, this position puts a complete stretch on almost the whole nervous system. If there is anything like a bit of disc pressing on the spinal cord, then it can't stretch as it should and there will be an increase in pain. So, if there is *no* increase in pain then we can start to rule out problems in the spine itself.

If the SLR is full range and pain free then there cannot be a problem with the mobility of the sciatic nerve ie there is nothing pinching on the nerve. If there was, then there would be pain down the nerve when we try to stretch it.

This is a relatively simple test, which when done correctly and completely, can save the NHS thousands of pounds in unnecessary MRI and X rays!

MOVEMENT IN THE NERVOUS SYSTEM

What is not common knowledge is that the nervous system has to be able to stretch and move with our arms, legs and bodies. If you think about it, all the nerves etc have to be able to stretch and move, otherwise we wouldn't be able to move at all. Every movement of our arms and legs etc would be painful as the tension is put on the nerves with the movement.

It is only in the relatively recent past that anyone considered the movement of the nervous system at all. Medical research has always been so busy looking for disease processes and what might kill us off, that the idea of pain being caused by the actual movement of nerves that are effectively "glued" at one end, was never really considered.

I well remember going on my first course in Neuro-orthopaedics back in the 1980's. It was a revelation! Suddenly so much slotted into place. This was the first time that I became aware of the fact that nerve impulses can travel in both directions

REFLEXES

This is the next stage in the examination process and for low back pain, we check three reflexes: the knee, the ankle and a rather odd one called the plantar response or Babinski response.

The knee reflex works through the 3rd lumbar nerve, with a bit of the 4th lumbar nerve. The ankle reflex works through the 5th lumbar and the 1st sacral nerve, and the plantar response can indicate possible serious pathology of the central nervous system ie the brain and spinal cord.

So what's going on here?

Reflexes are a test of a spinal reflex that happens when you stretch a tendon.

This means that the body has a safety mechanism designed to stop you over stretching the tendon attachment of the muscle to the bone. It is designed to stop the tendons being ripped off the bone as well as protecting the joint underneath.

IMPORTANT POINT 1

The body needs to protect its joints from damage. If the joints don't work properly then the whole body could be at risk. In other words, your body can't function. You might not be able to move to get food, or you may not be able to feed yourself – as well as many other required human activities!

There are little sensors in the tendons that fire off a signal to the spinal cord, which in turn fires back a message to the muscles to contract to stop any over stretching or damage to these soft tissues. This is an entirely automatic response. The reason why the messages go up to the spinal cord and back again is for speed. If it went all the way up to the brain where you have time to consciously think about what was going on, then it would be too late and the damage would be done before you realise it!

When we hit the tendon of the quadriceps muscle with a reflex hammer, just under the knee cap (patella), we are stretching that tendon and stimulating these little sensors to fire off to the spinal cord, which in turn sends the signal back to the quadriceps making them contract and straighten the knee. This happens in an instant if the system is working well.

IMPORTANT POINT 2

A good examination will include a number of tests for the same thing to back up, or not, the likelihood of a particular structure or condition being the problem. If the signs and symptoms do not fit the proposed hypotheses, then there should be no treatment offered until a definitive diagnosis has been made.
What is happening is that the doctor, or other healthcare practitioner, thinks that it may be this, or that, and tries different treatment options until something works. In other words, if a treatment seems to work then it must be that problem. This is a very dangerous way to work and serious diagnoses can be missed. I have seen this too often in medico-legal cases where diagnoses are missed because the GP did not have the time, or the detailed knowledge to make the right decisions.
Reflexes are a good example of this and not all healthcare practitioners "bother" with this essential testing for neurological issues.

The quadriceps muscle and the associated tendon are supplied by the femoral nerve that comes mainly from the 3rd lumbar nerve, with a bit from the 4th lumbar nerve. If the muscle doesn't't contract then we start thinking that something is interfering with the nerves from this level, or that we haven't carried out the test well enough, or the muscle can over-respond and a "brisk" contraction is seen. This can mean a number of things including the nerve being over sensitive.
The ankle reflex is where we hit the calf muscle tendon (gastrocnemius). This reflex tests the 5th lumbar and 1st sacral nerve. Again, if there is any abnormality in the reflex reaction then it indicates a possible problem at this level.

The Babinski, or plantar response is where we take the pointed end of the reflex hammer and scrape it up the sole of your foot – usually towards the little toe side. What should happen ie a normal response, is that the toes will bend down (go into flexion). In babies under about 3 months old, the toes go the other way, up into extension. If this response is seen in anyone over 3 months old, then we consider it a definite "red flag" situation that needs medical examination in the shape of scans, x rays and/or blood tests. Again we would be looking for other possible signs and symptoms that would support the possibility of serious pathology.

IMPORTANT POINT 3

Most people who get low back pain don't get muscle weakness as a result of pressure on a nerve. Of the people who do have muscle weakness there are even fewer who have weakness involving more than one nerve ie a more serious problem somewhere in the central nervous system.

Back to the examination:

MUSCLE POWER (MYOTOMES)

With you still lying on your back, the next aspect to look at is for any weakness in particular muscle groups supplied by the nerves to the legs. We've looked at the reflexes linked to the nerves, now we need to look at other structures supplied by these nerves – in this case the muscles.

What we do is to get you to work easily accessible muscles. If we select one muscle per nerve supply then if there is a problem with the nerve that is big enough to cause issues with the nerve supply to the muscles, then it will show up as weakness in that muscle.

For example, the quadriceps muscle is supplied by the 3rd lumbar nerve. So, if that nerve is affected enough, then there will be weakness in your ability to straighten your knee. If there is weakness in the quadriceps, then we will look for weakness in other muscle groups. We would look for weakness in other muscles supplied by the same nerve, as well as looking to see if other nerves are involved.

If the weakness is limited to the one nerve, then this would most commonly be a problem in the spine and or the sacro-iliac joints. If there is weakness involving more than one nerve, this suggests something could be affecting the central nervous system - the brain and spinal cord. Although this is rare, it is obviously important that such weakness is not missed.

How the spinal cord stretches

It is now well established that the spinal cord does not stretch like an elastic band. It has to stretch like the rest of the nervous system because our whole bodies move and stretch. When you bend down to touch your toes, the sciatic nerve has to stretch at least 2 inches to allow you to get down there. As a result it is more likely to be tightening of the nerve that stops you getting down there rather than tightness in the hamstrings on the back of the thigh - unless you happen to damage your hamstrings playing sport.

The only other factor to consider here is that we inherit 80% of our flexibility from our parents. So, if both your parents are not bendy, then you won't be either. On the other hand, if your mother can actually touch hers toes, then the likelihood is that you will be able to do that as well. If both your parents can touch their toes, then you will be able to do it too.

There is no right or wrong with this.

If you have never been able to touch your toes, then don't spend hours at the gym trying to get down to your toes, because you are only able to work on stretching the 20% of flexibility that you didn't inherit!

It is very definitely not a sign of fitness in being able to touch your toes!

The spinal cord stretches from 3 points along the spine. In the middle of the neck, it stretches up and down at the same time. This seems very counter-intuitive, but there is a good reason.

This stretching in both ways also happens in the middle of the thoracic spine (between the shoulder blades) and lumbar spine.

Touching toes with toes turned in or out. Hamstrings or Sciatic nerve?

A simple way of seeing whether it is your sciatic nerve or hamstrings that are stopping you touching your toes is to stand with your toes turned out and then bend down and touch them with your knees straight. Feel what stretch there is down your legs and how far you get. Now turn your toes in towards each other and repeat the touching toes. Again, feel what the stretch is like and how far you get.

Compare which version was easier. Could you reach further and with less stretch with your toes turned out, or with your toes turned in? The point here is that you are putting more stretch on the sciatic nerve with your toes turned in and more stretch on the hamstrings with your toes turned out.

This is why, when we do the Straight Leg Raise test, we turn your foot in and pull your toes up. This is literally winding up the sciatic nerve and if you think about it, it is the same movement whether you are lying on your back having your leg taken up into the straight leg position, your foot turned in and toes pulled up, and standing with your toes turned in and touching your toes. You either lift your leg up, or take your body down. It is the same movement. This is such an easy test to distinguish between tightness in the hamstrings or the sciatic nerve.

BLADDER RESPONSE S4 PALSY

This is a very important point for anyone who has low back pain.

If the pain is caused by problems with a disc in the low lumbar spine, then there is the possibility that the part of the disc could move far enough to seriously affect the spinal cord. If the disc material moves far enough backwards onto the spinal cord at this level, it can start interfering with the nerves that supply the sphincters of the bladder and/or bowel. This means that you start to lose the control and start to become incontinent.

If this happens, it is generally considered that the disc has to be removed within 48 hours or the loss of control of the sphincters may be permanent.

If this is the situation with someone you know, or yourself, then you must go to your doctor or the Accident and Emergency department at your local hospital and tell them that this has happened.

In a routine examination of the low back, this question should always be asked of the patient.

PALPATION

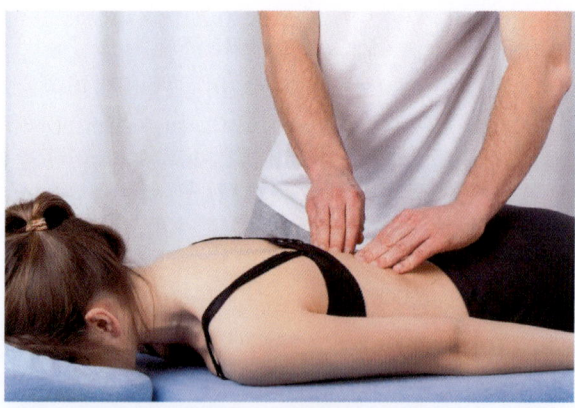

This means actually putting hands on you the patient! It cannot be done through clothes, and it cannot be done with you standing – it has to be carried out with you lying on your front on the examination couch.

The purpose of actually "prodding and poking" your back varies a little with the examiner and their particular training and preference.

Generally, we are looking and feeling for anything that is out of the ordinary. This means looking for symmetry in the spinous processes (the bony bits that stick directly backwards from the vertebral bodies), feeling how deep the spinous process of the last lumbar vertebra (L5) is from the base of the sacrum. If there is a big drop off the sacral base to the L5 spinous process, then we start thinking about a condition called spondylolisthesis. This is where the L5 vertebra has moved forward slightly on the sacral base.

There are 5 grades of slip and the worst possible, but very rare situation is where the vertebra could go through the spinal cord sitting in the middle. This would result in paralysis of the body from the waist down. This would have the same effect as breaking your back! Of course this situation is very rare and usually only happens following severe trauma to the back. We would know about any trauma from the Subjective history and our examination so far!

The lesser grades happen as a result of problems with the ligaments, or the small joints on either side of the vertebra (facet joints). This means that the segment, or spinal level, has become unstable structurally. Grades 1 and 2 can be treated conservatively with very specific stabilising exercises and techniques, but Grades 3 to 5 really need a surgical operation to fix that segment with bone grafts and/or screws to stop the vertebra moving.

Palpation is also a way of identifying any increased tone, or tension in the muscles of either side of the spine. It requires a great deal of skill to find these abnormalities and just because you have a degree in physiotherapy or medicine, does not mean that you are experienced enough to identify these possible abnormalities!

Some people tend to look for painful areas only. My view is that you can find tender points anywhere, on anybody – if you poke hard enough! Just because there is a tender point does not necessarily mean that the problem lies under the skin just where you have pushed. Of course, there are times when this is exactly right, but that tender point needs to be backed up by other positive signs and symptoms, otherwise it is an isolated feature.

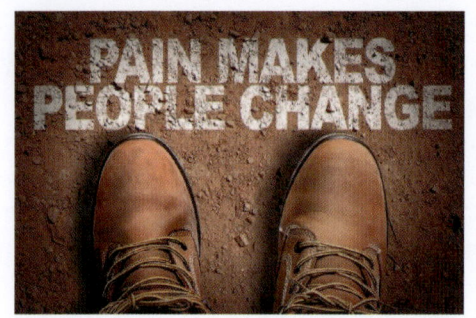

Persistent pain from another source can also "sensitise" the nervous system so that a little bit of pressure with a finger actually becomes painful from the patient's point of view. But, more of that later.

Chapter 4

THE DIAGNOSIS

So what can we learn from all this information that we have gathered from the objective examination?

To make sense of all this, we need to have a good knowledge of the anatomy of the area and just how things work and move!

I can make this very complicated, but I think it can be very easily explained:

There are 3 sets of joints that could cause the problem of low back pain. These are:

The **inter-vertebral joints** with the disc between.
The **facet joints** on either side of the intervertebral joints.
The **sacro-iliac joints** sitting below the spine and in the ring of the pelvis.

The point here is that there are no other joints in the area.

There are the ligaments that hold the joints together, the muscles that stabilise the joints and the muscles that move the joints. There are the nerves that supply the joints and the blood vessels and lymphatics that flow into and out of the area. There are sundry other soft tissues, but they are there to make the joints work and move so that you can work and move.

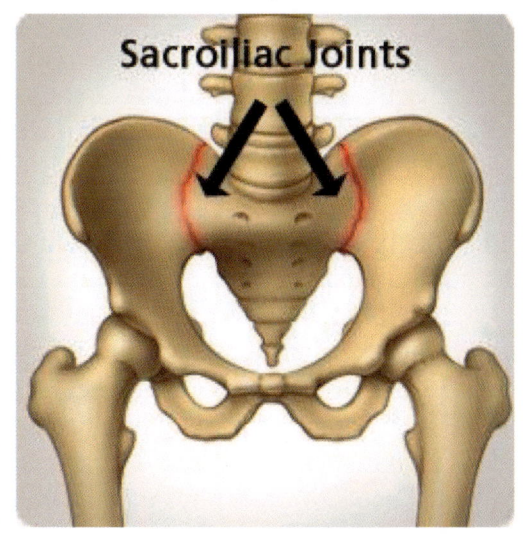

It seems to me that to have an injury to say one muscle on its own is impossible. I do not see how one small component of a complex and integrated system, can be injured without damage to its neighbouring structures. I can definitely understand how a *joint* can be damaged, which in turn will affect part or all of the associated soft tissues, but not the other way around.

Of course, this is not including diseases. I am talking about simple low back pain which is not functioning because of a mechanical problem. Maybe the answer is in the name? "Simple low back pain" is also called "mechanical low back pain". This label has been used by doctors, physiotherapists and others for many years now, but still there is the idea that no-one knows what causes the problems, or how to treat them effectively. Surely the answer is in the name? Mechanical low back pain says there is a problem with the mechanics of the back – and in my book at least, this has to be the joints first!

I suggest that the thought that it has to be a muscle injury came about because doctors couldn't find a disease process that would fit the picture presented by patients with low back pain. So, they thought it had to be caused by a problem in the musculo-skeletal system. The thinking, or clinical reasoning was right but the knowledge wasn't there to really identify the cause of the pain, because medical students are not taught to examine or treat musculo-skeletal conditions in any great depth.

This is why there are post graduate courses in musculo-skeletal medicine for both doctors and physiotherapists. The Society of Musculoskeletal Medicine (SOMM) is the only organisation that runs post graduate courses for both doctors and physiotherapists. Until recently it was called the Society of Orthopaedic Medicine, but the term "musculoskeletal medicine" has become the standard term for all those conditions that affect the skeleton and the structures that make it move.

Physiotherapy is the leading profession for the diagnosis and treatment of musculoskeletal conditions, but as with doctors, you need to find physiotherapists who have specialised in this area. Not all physiotherapists are the same with the same set of skills and expertise, any more than all doctors are the same. You wouldn't go to a gynaecologist with a broken leg, so don't go to a neuro-physiotherapist with low back pain! Equally, if you need rehabilitation following a stroke, then don't go to a physiotherapist whose specialist skills are in musculoskeletal medicine.

So what can go wrong with these joints?

THE INTERVERTEBRAL JOINTS

In the lumbar spine, the intervertebral discs can be loaded and eventually fail – to a greater or lesser extent.

The discs are made up of a tough outer "shell" – the annulus, and a softer inside – the nucleus.

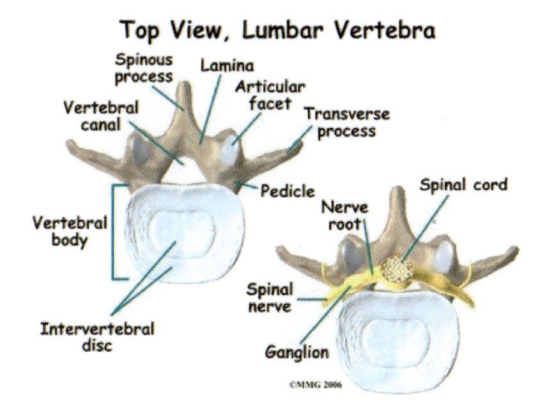

From this diagram, you can see how the disc sits in front of the spinal cord and the spinal nerves. So if any bits of the disc, such as small sections of the annulus, break off then they could move backwards onto the spinal cord – causing back pain, or slightly sideways onto the spinal nerve – causing pain into the buttock and the leg.

Cracks, or small splits can appear in the annulus with age and wear and tear, and this then gives the soft nucleus a route through to the sensitive cord and spinal nerves.

This does not answer the question of back pain in children!

It should be noted that the whole disc doesn't "slip". It is very firmly attached to the bodies of the vertebrae above and below. So the old diagnosis of "slipped disc" is not accurate. Neither does the annulus fragment like a digestive biscuit!

The action of bending forward effectively "opens" the back of the vertebra and "closes" the front of the joint. If any bit of the disc is going to move, then by bending the back you are encouraging disc material to move towards the spinal cord and nerves.

THE FACET JOINTS

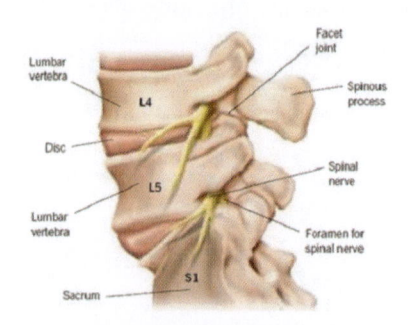

The facet joints can be strained and then "screwed down" by the tightening of the surrounding protective muscle spasm

This tightening down of the facet joints can cause increased pressure on the discs, but the most common problem is the effective narrowing of the space between the facet joints on the side of the spine where the spinal nerves emerge. If the spinal nerve is squashed as it comes off the spinal cord, there will be pain down the leg

Low back pain is virtually never caused by muscle injury, except where there is direct injury or trauma.

What is also commonly missed is the fact that simply half bending over the wash hand basin to clean your teeth, loads the low back with 2/3 of your body weight. In other words the joints of the low back are loaded with this additional weight and if they cannot take that strain then you feel pain with the disruption of the joints of the spine.

I want to give you an understanding of the anatomy of the spine and pelvis so that you can begin to realise what is going on when you get back pain. For any health professionals who may be reading this book, I make no apologies for the simplicity of this chapter as my intention is to demystify the whole problem.

By stripping the anatomy back to basics then you can begin to see where the problems may lie. What I am also going to do is to combine the what is known about disease processes, mechanisms of injury and how the body takes and manages loading with changes in muscle activity leading to changes in movement patterns. What this does is to combine the core knowledge of doctors and physiotherapists.

Doctors are not generally aware of the huge amount of research that goes on in the physiotherapy profession around the world as what we are looking at is the intricate mechanisms of how the body actually moves, what happens when this mechanism goes wrong and how to restore normal movement patterns. Doctors are looking at cell level for disease processes and how to treat or manage them.

THE ANATOMY

The spine is made up of 24 blocks stacked on top of one another. These are the vertebrae. There are seven in the neck (cervical spine), twelve in the mid back (thoracic spine) and 5 in the low back (lumbar spine). These building blocks of the spine are essentially the same at all levels, but with certain differences that reflect the needs of movement and function at the different levels.

The cervical spine vertebrae are smaller than the thoracic spine and the largest of all are the lumber spine vertebrae.

The lumbar spine vertebrae take far more load as they have to support the weight and movement of the whole of the body above the waist. The cervical spine, on the other hand, needs to move far more because we want to move our heads, which weigh about 10 pounds.

The size of the vertebrae are smaller and the neck is far more flexible. The thoracic spine has the 12 pairs of ribs attached, which in turn are there to protect the lungs, heart etc by forming a cage around the internal organs. The range of movement at this level is less than in the cervical spine but more than in the lumbar spine.

You can see that each section has a different function and corresponding movement pattern.

Normal Spine

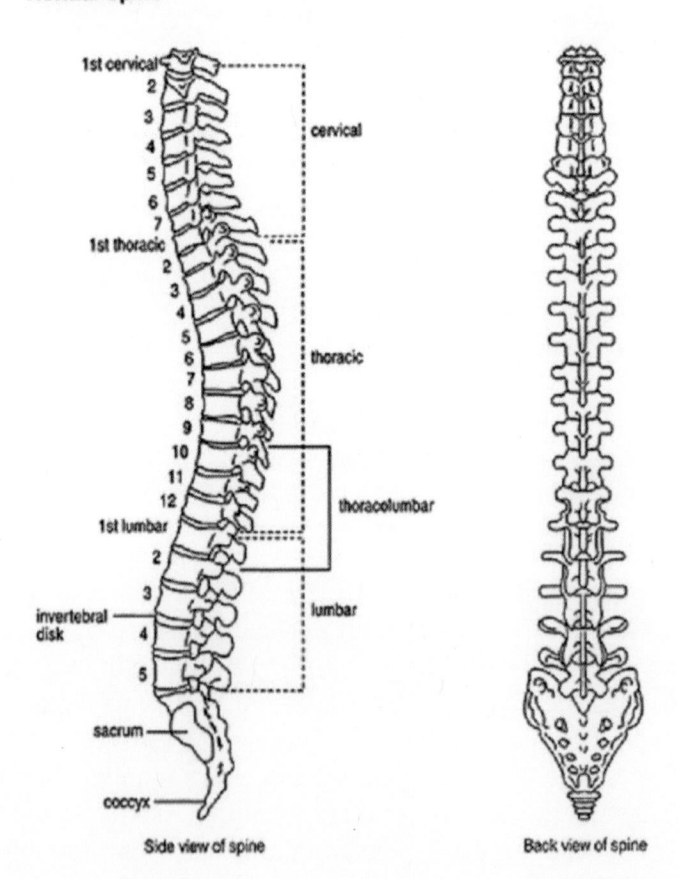

Next comes the curves of the spine and there are a lot of different opinions about these and a lot of mis-information. Simply, in the womb, the whole spine is curved forward.

After birth, and as the baby develops into being able to stand upright on two feet, the lumbar spine develops a curve, the thoracic spine then curves the opposite way and the neck curves the same way as the lumbar spine. This is what gives the whole spine the S shape.

If the spine was simply a straight rod, then there would be no capacity to take the shock and compression forces of walking and running on 2 feet rather than 4.

There is another consideration when thinking about the curves in the spine, which is the position of the sacrum that lies below the lumbar spine and within the ring of the pelvis. The sacrum is the foundation of the spine and sits in the ring of the pelvis in a position where it is slightly tipped forwards.

If the spine followed this angle, then we would stand tipped forwards at about 45 degrees. In order to stand upright, there has to be this backward curve – the other way in the lumbar spine; with a corresponding forward curve in the thoracic spine, and another backward curve in the cervical spine to keep the head upright so we can see where we are going.

These are the natural curves of the spine. The hollow in the lumbar spine needs to be kept regardless of what position we are in. This means that if we bend forwards to pick something up from the floor, then the correct way to do this is to bend from the hips.

The spine sits on top of the sacrum, and the coccyx or tailbone is the small residual "tail" attached underneath the sacrum.

If the mechanical loading through the spine is altered, then stresses and strains can happen and the joints of the spine can either fail or eventually become arthritic.

The sacrum works like the keystone in the arch. We now know that the sacrum moves in the opposite direction to the spine above.

If you bend down to touch your toes, the sacrum tips backwards underneath it. Equally, of you bend backwards - arching your spine, the sacrum will tip forwards.

It used to be thought that the sacral joints only moved, or loosened a week to ten days before periods, or during childbirth. It was thought that these joints didn't move at all in men and only occasionally in women.

With dynamic ultrasound scanning, the actual movement of the joints could be seen and it was shown that the sacrum could move up to 1cm.

If this movement did not exist between the sacrum and the pelvis; the sacrum and the spine, and the pelvis bones in the front (the pubic symphysis) there would be no shock absorbing system.

In other words, if you jumped off a kerb, then with no movement in the system, the bones would have to take the load and probably fracture.

There is a similar situation in the bones of the skull. The suture lines between the bones of the skull take up the shock forces to prevent you cracking, or fracturing your skull every time you hit your head. By the time we reach 80 years old, then these suture lines are effectively fused, and the risk of fracturing the bones of the skull if we fall over is very real.

The spinal cord finishes at the second lumbar vertebra. Below that, there is a collection of spinal nerves that travel down within the spine, coming out on either side of the remaining vertebrae and through holes on either side of the sacrum.

Without this co-ordinated activity of the muscles and joints concerned, then pain, disability, dysfunction and maladaption, or abnormal movement, will happen. Let's not forget the nerves in all this.

SACRO-ILIAC DYSFUNCTIONS

It is now a well established and researched fact

that as we walk or run the bones of the pelvis rotate and move up and down.

Over the last 10 years, dynamic ultrasound scans and examinations principally by the American physiotherapists have shown that there can be about 30 dysfunctions in and around this area.

Your spine and pelvis form the foundations of your whole body. If the foundations are not set correctly, the house will fall down!

In its simplest form, if your posture is not good then you will get aches and pains involving many and various joints because they are being used and loaded in an abnormal way.

Look at this picture:

The two sides of the pelvis, the sacrum and lumbar spine all work together as a unit. The muscles that work this unit must do so in a very specific and interactive way. Without this co-ordinated activity of the right muscles and joints, then pain, disability, dysfunction and maladaption, or abnormal movements, can happen.

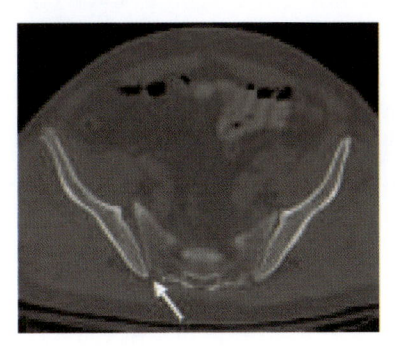

Seemingly simply injuries and accidents can upset the balance of this mechanism and lie dormant for many years. Then you sneeze, or bend slightly awkwardly, and the whole system falls apart causing pain and dysfunction.

THEIR POSSIBLE EFFECTS

These scans are a cross section of the sacro-iliac joints. You can see clearly the asymmetry between the pelvis bones and the sacrum in the middle. The "face" in the middle of the scans is the sacrum bone and the "wings" are the pelvis bones. They should be equal on both sides and not showing the differences between left and right as in these pictures.

If the sacropelvic region of the pelvis fails to function correctly, then there will be knock-on effects. These can be reflected up the spine causing disc degeneration, rib dysfunctions, neck and shoulder problems, headaches and even migraines.

There can also be problems reflected down into the legs and feet. These can be altered "tracking" and weight transmission through the hips, knees and feet, which may lead ultimately to arthritis.

Before the onset of such joint disease there is likely to be marked changes in the efficient use of the legs. If the weight transmission through the legs is altered then the muscles can't function efficiently.

HOW DOES THIS HAPPEN?

Sudden twisting or bending movements can cause problems of this type. Falling over, or accidents, are the obvious culprits, but even slipping and not quite falling over commonly causes problems.

A mild problem with the sacro-pelvic joints can happen without being noticed until some time later when sufficient load is put on the joints again and the problem is then enough to cause pain and difficulties in moving around.

POSSIBLE CAUSES

There is a school of thought that says that we are not really designed to sit on chairs.

Sitting puts us into a fixed and unnatural position that can load the sacro-iliac joints and the lumbar spine. If we sit too long, muscles may shorten in such a way that when we stand up the pelvis is always tilted too far forwards. This in turn loads small joints on either side of the spine.

These conditions are not visible on Xray or conventional scans. These are problems that affect one bone attempting to move against another.

A detailed clinical examination is designed to find the exact problem. It has to be a dynamic/motion-testing one, and it has to be carried out by specialist, chartered physiotherapists who have the necessary post-graduate training and skill.

By going through a series of movements and palpating the joints as the motion is carried out, the physiotherapist can tell exactly which dysfunction is present.

Accurate diagnosis is essential. As physiotherapists, we look for specific tissues that may be at fault, but we also look for possible problems in the HUMAN MOVEMENT SYSTEM. This is the area that is the specific province of physiotherapists.

It is possible to have problems with the human movement system and for your pain to come from these problems and not from a specific tissue.

WHAT CAN BE DONE?

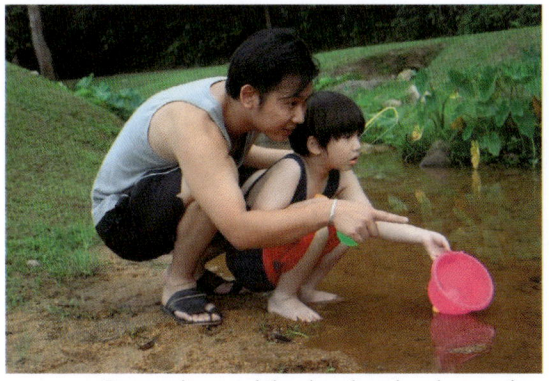

Exercises which help to maintain the flexibility of the body are so important to keep the function and efficiency of the body's movement. - especially in competitive sport.

Squatting with the heels down is one of the most useful exercises - in that it "opens" the sacro-iliac joints and allows them to return to the normal position.

PHYSIOTHERAPY

Contrary to what you might still read in dictionaries or even in Back Care books sponsored by certain chemist chains, physiotherapy treatment may involve manipulation, mobilisations, or myotactic activation procedures (MAP's). All these techniques are designed to move the bones of the pelvis back into the correct working position.

This is no problem to the expert practitioner, but what is needed afterwards is the re-training of the stabilising muscle system that needs to be working efficiently - both from the strength and timing viewpoint, in order to restore the normal function and maintenance of the whole system.

This rehabilitation process brings in the work of the Australian physiotherapists who have carried out enormous amounts of research into the stabilising muscle systems.

They have also established the mechanisms involved in restoring the stabilisers of the neck in whiplash injuries. The same principles apply.

See the work of Prof Paul Hodges, Prof Gwen Jull, Mark Comerford et al on Google.

It constantly amazes me that there is still a significant part of the population that are completely unaware that Physiotherapy is a profession (not a treatment) that is more than 120 years old and requires a university degree ie at least a BSc honours degree in Physiotherapy.

Professor Paul Hodges has 3 PhDs – one in Physiotherapy and two in Neuroscience!

THE CORE MUSCLES

Core Stability describes the body's ability to control the trunk. This is an interaction between the way we are built, our muscles' ability to work and the way our brains work our muscles.

The stabilisers don't fatigue easily, they work at a low intensity and stay activated for long periods of time. The stabilisers are important for maintaining posture and preventing injury by finely controlling the position of the body in space.

The Deep stabilising muscles of the trunk include:

1. Transversus abdominis
2. Deep fibres of multifidus
3. Pelvic floor
4. Diaphragm

GOOD MUSCLE FUNCTION

The deep stabilising muscles of the trunk form a muscular cylinder surrounding the lumbar spine and pelvis. The deep stabilisers help control the position and movement of the trunk. The mover muscles are more superficial, they are the muscles you use to move your body.

THE DEEP STABILISER MUSCLES

1. Work at low intensity for long periods of time
2. Generate tension to support and stabilise rather than move the body
3. Contract before you move to support the body's position
4. Turn on in a similar way no matter what way you are moving
5. Keep the spine and pelvis optimally aligned to maintain a neutral spine or 'good posture' position.

THE MUSCLES THAT MOVE THE JOINTS

1. Work at high intensity for short periods of time
2. Generate force to move the body and change its position
3. Contract to cause the movement of the trunk and limbs
4. Work differently depending on which movement you are doing.

The deep stabiliser muscles only work at about 5% of their maximal contraction, but stay on for long periods of time. As they contract, the stabilisers don't move your body much, if at all. They tend to apply tension and support structures rather than move your body.

When you think of moving, the deep stabilisers contract before any of the muscles that actually cause the movement. This pre-contraction prepares your body for the movement by supporting and stabilising the trunk to provide a stable base for movement.

A stable base makes for mechanically efficient movement or static postures.

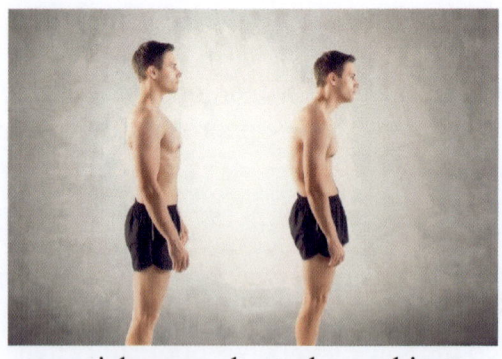

Imagine a crane being positioned on a solid concrete slab versus a sandy beach.

The crane on the concrete slab is much more easily controlled by the driver who can be more accurate as the crane picks up and sets down objects.

The crane on the beach will be much less accurate and take more effort getting the objects placed exactly where it wants them. This in turn will reduce sporting performance as well as making everyday activities increasingly difficult.

The deep stabilising muscles of the body provide the stable base (concrete slab) for the mover muscles to move the trunk and limbs.

WHAT ABOUT SCIATICA?

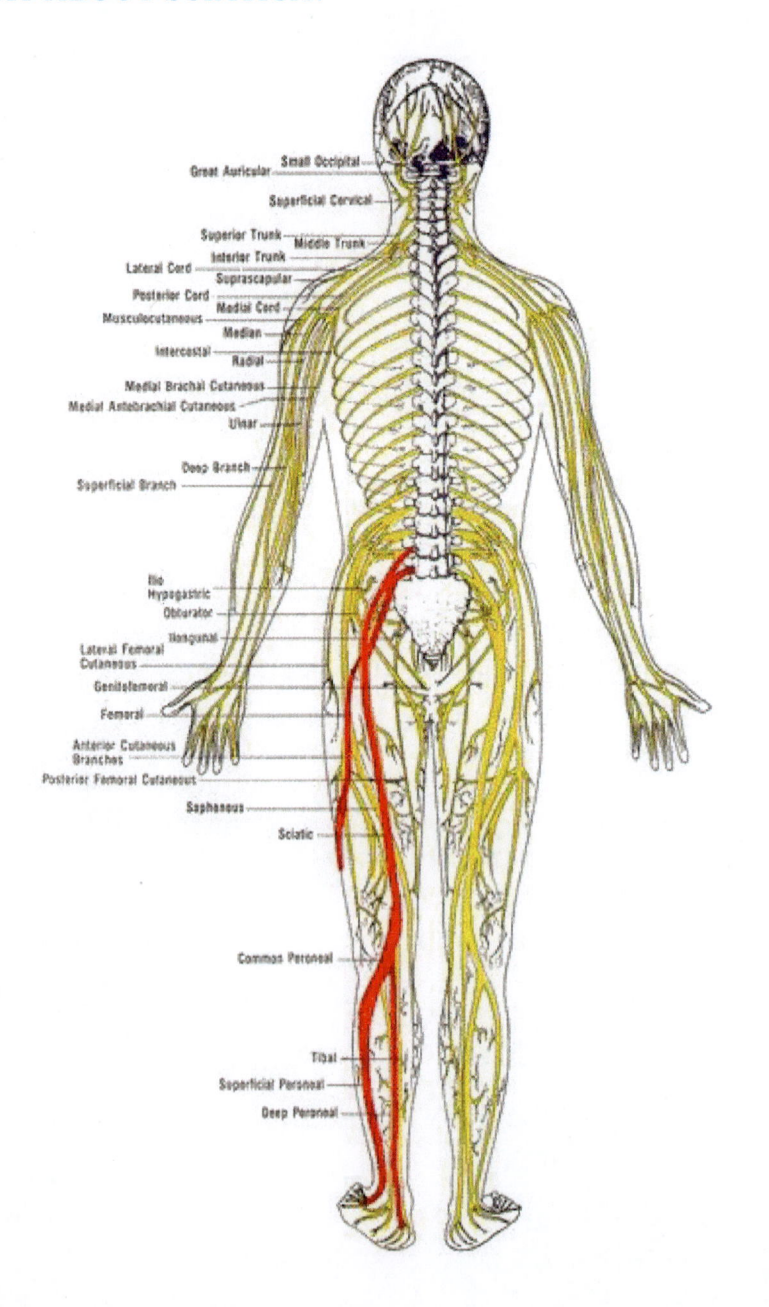

The sciatic nerve is the largest nerve in the body. It is made up of nerves that come out of the side of the last two lumbar vertebrae and out of the 4 holes of either side of the sacrum.

Parts of the sciatic nerve can be squashed at different levels, and this is what gives a different pain and disability picture with different conditions.

True sciatica is usually caused by part of a disc squashing a branch of the sciatic nerve against part of the vertebra.

The term "sciatica" is a symptom, not a diagnosis!

It describes pain down the leg - it does not explain the reason for the pain in the leg. This pain is like a searing knife down the leg. It is constant and does not come and go.

Pain that is aching in character; that varies in how far down the leg it goes and varies in intensity depending on activity, is not true sciatica. It is probably caused by the nerve, or part of it, being stretched and irritated as it passes through the pelvis.

WHAT ELSE CAN CAUSE PAIN IN THE LEG?

"Gentle" pressure on the sciatic nerve usually happens when the piriformis muscle tightens up as a result of a sacral dysfunction. This muscle comes from the front of the sacrum (one on either side) goes through the pelvis, and attaches onto the bony lump on the side of the hip (greater trochanter).

This produces a deep, nebulous sort of pain that aches down the side of the leg. It is not sharp and it comes and goes without apparent cause.

As a general rule, the further down the leg the pain goes, the more pressure and even damage, to the nerve has occurred.

The exact distribution and character of the pain tells us the most likely cause and origin of the problem. Just to complicate things, there can be more than one problem causing similar symptoms.

This is why we use a number of clinical tests designed to test each possible structure that could cause the symptoms.

For example, pain down the front of the leg may be caused by hip joint problems or irritation of the femoral nerve that comes off the spinal cord at the level of the 3rd lumbar vertebra.

So, we test both structures to see which is causing the pain.

If this clinical test shows a significant problem with the hip joint itself, then tests such as X rays and scans may be needed to decide the best course of action.

Chapter 5

TREATMENT FOR LOW BACK PAIN

Before consenting to any treatment it is vital to understand just what the treatment involves and the expected outcome.

I'm going to explain the detail of the most commonly used treatments, their benefits and any possible side effects. These treatments may be offered by physiotherapists, osteopaths, Chiropractors, Sports therapists and masseurs.

I will list some of the options offered by orthopaedic surgeons, rheumatologists and GPS, but the detail of any procedures or medications will be for you to discuss with the doctor, as these are outside of my remit as a physiotherapist.

I will give you some indication of their uses, but I would urge you to keep asking questions about them until you really understand what the benefits and risks are. This of course applies to physical treatments as well as surgical options and medications.

MANIPULATION

Manipulation is just one therapeutic technique that comes under the general banner of "manual therapy".

It is technically a high velocity, low amplitude thrust technique that is specifically designed to loosen joints, or to move loose bodies within joints. It is a *passive* movement in that it is a technique carried out on the patient who essentially just needs to lie there - and keep breathing!

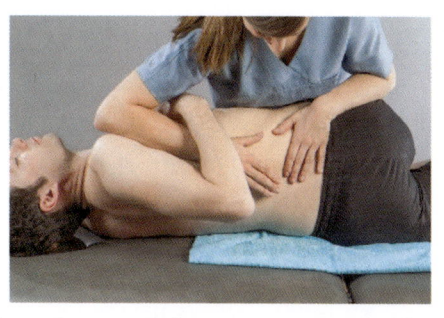

Correct manipulation means taking a joint to the end of its available range and applying a small, quick movement to take the joint that small bit further.

This picture is not how we manipulate people today! It is a picture showing manipulation with traction that was used as a treatment in Turkey in 1465.

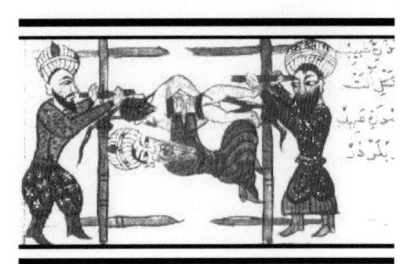

Today it is used principally by physiotherapists, osteopaths and chiropractors, but it has its roots in traditional medicine and by various cultures and for thousands of years. Hippocrates, the "father of medicine" apparently used manipulation as did the ancient Egyptians and many other cultures. So it is not new!

I have used it virtually every day of my professional life since I completed Dr Cyriax' course in Orthopaedic Medicine in 1978. I have found it to be one of the most useful techniques for my patients, but the medical community cannot really make up its mind about the efficacy and value particularly in the treatment of low back and neck pain. There have been many studies into manipulation that are overall inconclusive.

Part of the problem is that manipulation is a generic term that covers many different styles and systems depending on training and profession. There are some similarities in these techniques largely because there are only so many ways that you can actually move a joint, and this is specific to the individual joints. It varies with the anatomy and biomechanics of the joints. Physiotherapists, osteopaths and chiropractors approach the problem of back pain from different perspectives. Physiotherapists and osteopaths are probably the closest in their approach, but the chiropractors have a different ethos underpinning their clinical reasoning and techniques.

Manipulation is taught in training as a standard treatment to osteopaths and chiropractors, whereas there are relatively few physiotherapists who learn these techniques at a post graduate level, because the whole profession is split into different specialisms - in the same way as medicine. So only those of us who have specialised in MSK conditions have the need to learn these highly specialised techniques.

I suggest that it is these differences in manipulation techniques that have not been fully appreciated by the researchers. The other point to remember is the variation in clinical reasoning for using manipulation. Following the Orthopaedic Medicine approach devised by Dr Cyriax, we carry out manipulation only when it is absolutely necessary and it forms part of the whole treatment "recipe". This is because repeated, say weekly, manipulations can cause stretching and even damage to the ligaments that hold the joints together. If this happens, then it can make the spinal joints unstable and liable to even more damage. In very extreme cases, it can lead to paralysis and permanent disability.

Manipulation of the neck joints can even cause death by damaging the blood vessels that go up through the bones of the neck to the brain, causing stroke. To put it into proportion, it is estimated that serious damage following manipulation of the neck occurs in about 0.25 to 2 in a million. No deaths have occurred following manipulation by physiotherapists.

We should not forget that there is also the possibility of complications following surgery and there are all the known side effects of medication. So always be sure of the qualifications and experience of any healthcare professional that you go to see.

I don't manipulate low backs in exactly the same way that I was taught by Dr Cyriax, because over the years I have adapted the techniques to suit what I can physically manage. Also, I have reduced the amount of force that I use, because with 40+ years of experience in handling and moving patient's spines, I can be far more subtle about the range of movement I need. I like to work on the principle of the least amount of force needed to achieve the required result!

This illustrates the point! This is what makes research and surveys very difficult. Physical treatments like manipulation are not drug doses. There are too many variables - the diagnosis (if any was made), the patient **and** the healthcare practitioner.

It is not possible to do so called "sham" manipulations, because it is a treatment that the patient **feels** and is physically aware of! It is not like giving people pills, with no active ingredient, where they don't know if they are taking an active drug, or whether they belong to the placebo group as a control.

SHORT PERSONAL STORY:

As an illustration of this, I will to tell you about a personal experience I had when I was Superintendent Physiotherapist working at St Bartholomew's Hospital in London back in the late 1970s.

My husband and I lived in Great Dunmow, Essex and we both worked in central London. We would drive into London every day down the M11. In those days if there were more than 2 cars on the motorway then it was a traffic jam!

This particular day, I went to sleep during the drive (I wasn't driving, my husband was!). When we got to Barts, I couldn't move my neck because of all the bouncing around the back turnings in East London!

I spent almost the entire day going from A and E for an X ray, to the Mobilisation Unit of the Physiotherapy Department for traction and mobilisations and back to my office for a sit down with a large cup of coffee! By 5pm I was still in a lot of pain and still couldn't move my neck.

By this time I was really getting frustrated and I grabbed one of my senior physiotherapists who I knew trained at St Thomas" Hospital, London in the days when Dr Cyriax used to teach the student physiotherapists about Orthopaedic Medicine and his manipulation techniques.

Within 10 minutes, she had done a quick examination, because we both knew what the problem was, and she had manipulated my neck. I had almost no pain and full range of movement in my neck. Within 2 hours, I was back to normal.

To sum up this discussion, I know that whatever the precise, physiological action of manipulation, I have had literally thousands of patients where manipulation restores the range of movement and reduces the pain in a matter of moments. Of course there is still the need to reduce the inflammation and get back the normal muscle balance ie the rehabilitation element, but if we can see patients within the first 6 days of the onset of their back pain, then we can relieve the pain, restore the movement and get them back to work within days.

I am fully aware of the confirmed unbelievers out there, including doctors and other physiotherapists, but I would suggest that they have become so used to seeing people who have had low back pain for more than 6 weeks.

These are the patients who have had to wait months to see a physiotherapist on the NHS, or who have been taking the painkillers and anti-inflammatories for the past 2 months with very little real benefit.

These patients are then developing all the signs of a chronic condition. They are worried, concerned and fearful that they may lose their jobs, their homes etc and that this back pain is never going to go away!

They don't have enough information to see that there is a way out of this dilemma and a whole bunch of secondary issues and problems - both physiological and psychological, start to develop.

These patients need a different approach and manipulation is very unlikely to answer all of their problems, but it may form a part of the whole package.

One of the key points about manipulation is knowing when NOT to do it!

Any healthcare practitioner should know all the occasions when manipulation is contra-indicated. The key indicators simply remembered by COINS:

1. Circulatory disorders
2. Osteoporosis

3. Inflammatory conditions such as Rheumatoid arthritis
4. Neurological conditions
5. Serious pathology such as cancer

More specifically for low back pain, they are:

Bladder and bowel symptoms - because severe pressure on the spinal cord can interfere with the nerves that supply the sphincters of the bladder and bowel - the S4 palsy. This could be severe "slipped disc" or spinal tumours/ secondaries.

Saddle anaesthesia - this wonderfully historic phrase concerns any loss of sensation in those parts that would be in contact with the saddle of a horse were you sitting on it! Again it could be caused by severe pressure on the spinal cord itself.

Anticoagulant therapy - as the increased likelihood of bleeding can be a problem if blood vessels are damaged during the procedure.

Blood clotting disorders - same discussion as above, with haemophilia for example.

Inflammatory arthritis - where the joints are already inflamed, very sensitive and prone to damage.

Past history of trauma - there may be pre-existing fractures in bones from accidents or injuries that could be made worse with manipulation.

Past medical conditions - this in particular is where medical knowledge is necessary to understand the possible conditions that would make manipulation unsafe. Doctors and physiotherapists train within the NHS and have this knowledge. Healthcare practitioners who do not have this within their training may not have seen, or even know about these conditions.

Medications - the most obvious one in this category are the oral steroids that can cause osteoporosis, causing the bones to become brittle and likely to fracture with the additional force of manipulation.

General health - all sorts of conditions come under this heading, but I would also include those patients who have a fear of being manipulated. This is often overlooked as being a minor problem, but there are patients who are genuinely frightened about the whole process.

There are those patients we can bounce off the walls a few times and they will jump up and say that everything is better, but there are others who are terrified and see it as a physical assault. Whatever the origin of these fears, there is no doubt that these patients should be taken very seriously and their wishes respected.

But, particularly in physiotherapy, we have more tools in our "treatment box" and although it may take longer, there are lots of ways of dealing with the situation.

There are also times when manipulation can be carried out, but with caution! Whether manipulation is used is dependent on the skill, experience and knowledge of the healthcare practitioner and the probability of causing more harm than good. It requires a detailed discussion with the patient, and parent/guardian if under 16 years old, to decide on all the options and to have the right informed consent to proceed.

MOBILISATIONS

Mobilisations, or Maitland Mobilisations, were originally the work of an Australian Physiotherapist Geoff Maitland who pioneered the use of mobilisation for pain modulation. His models for practice and his descriptions for examination and treatment techniques are still taught today at undergraduate level to physiotherapists worldwide.

In 1965 he presented the first 3 month course on Manipulation of the Spine in Australia, and this subsequently developed into a full Master degree course. In 1974, he co-founded the International Federation of Orthopaedic Manipulative Therapy (IFOMPT), a branch of the World Confederation of Physiotherapy (WCPT). In 1981 he was awarded an MBE for his work and he is considered one of the great pioneers of physiotherapy.

From Geoff Maitland's book, Vertebral Manipulation, he describes the difference between mobilisation and manipulation:

"There are two ways of manipulating the conscious patient. The first, better thought of as mobilisation, is the gentle coaching of a movement by passive rhythmical oscillations performed within the limit of the range; the second is the forcing of a movement from the limit of the range by a sudden small thrust. The difference between these two techniques may seem negligible when comparing a strongly applied mobilisation with a gentle manipulative thrust, but there is an important difference. The patient can always resist the mobilisation if it should become too painful, whereas the suddenness of the forceful manipulation prevents any control by the patient."

The Maitland approach is different from Dr Cyriax' Orthopaedic Medicine concepts and maybe highlights some of the differences between doctors and physiotherapists. In practice, I think it better to have the best of both worlds for the benefit of the patient. What I mean is that for those patients whom we cannot manipulate, for whatever reason, we can use mobilisations. It is also a useful technique for getting the last few degrees of movement if necessary following manipulation. We also know that small amplitude mobilisations will stimulate the mechanoreceptors in the body, thereby giving pain relief

ELECTROTHERAPY

Electrotherapy today remains one of the four pillars of the scope of practice of the Physiotherapy Profession, as defined under our 1920 Royal Charter.

However. Over the last 15 to 20 years, electrotherapy generally has "fallen out of fashion" and is barely being taught in the universities today. To give you an idea, when I trained in the early 1970s, we had to learn the circuit diagrams of all the machines we used, even though we weren't allowed to change a plug in the hospital! We learnt how to apply many and various electrical currents for all sorts of conditions; all about ultra-violet lamps for the treatment of skin conditions, wounds and ulcers; how to apply heat with heat lamps and short wave diathermy and how to repair injuries with ultrasound and Interferential Therapy.

It was once said to me by a bioengineer that physiotherapists use almost every section of the electromagnetic spectrum, and he wasn't far wrong! I have a 1940s textbook on electrotherapy when they used even more techniques! One spectacular treatment was to put the patient into a bath of warm water, which had been isolated from earth. Then they put 4 electrodes into the water and passed a direct current through the patient in the bath. This was a treatment used for obesity, heart disease and general malaise, but they were more concerned that the patient might catch a chill from having to undress than they were about the near electrocution! Fortunately for the Professional Indemnity insurers we don't use most of these treatments any more.

There are two main reasons why there has been this decline in the use of electrotherapy:

The increasing demand for evidence based practice in all areas of healthcare has led to the universities refuting the benefits of electrotherapy in general, despite a great deal of research and evidence supporting Interferential Therapy (IFT) and ultrasound in particular.

This has led to the great reduction in teaching of the clinical application of all electrotherapy as part of the university curriculum.

I first really became involved with IFT in the late 1970s with the team of Bioengineers at Barts Hospital, London. This was the team that made the first British machine. I was asked to put in the "consumer" end for that machine and its successor.

I have worked with IFT ever since and carried out more than 100,000 treatments. It is an essential part of our treatment for low back pain as well as many other conditions. I seldom use it for pain relief!

I have also written a textbook on IFT and have the second revision to finish this year.

When we have the next generation of clinic machines, I will return to lecturing to physiotherapists on the wide range of clinical techniques and effects that can be achieved using IFT.

IFT is now only taught, and largely used, for pain relief.

University courses require any quoted research references to be less than 5 years. Therefore, all the research into IFT is now considered "out of date" and there are few physiotherapists aware of the amount of evidence that is actually available concerning the huge benefits of IFT as a treatment system.

A LITTLE HISTORY OF IFT

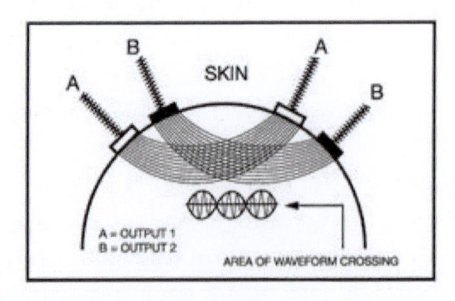

IFT was developed in Austria by Dr Nemec in the late 1940's. In 1949 the first machines were introduced into the UK and in 1979 the first British designed and manufactured machines were developed by the Bioengineering Department, in conjunction with the Physiotherapy Department, at St Bartholomew's Hospital, London.

The original Nemectrodyn IFT machines were limited in the frequency ranges produced and yet a great deal of research demonstrating the positive effects was carried out in the 1980's. Prof Lilyana Nikolova, in Bulgaria carried out a wide range of research – both on laboratory animals, and on human subjects. This research demonstrated that IFT will increase the healing rate of fractures and nerves, as well as showing beneficial effects on conditions of the internal organs and musculo-skeletal disorders.

The development of the British machines allowed for a wider range of frequency selection as well as far easier clinical applications. These machines became the leading devices in the electrotherapy field in the UK with sales starting to extend into Europe, Africa and the USA. Together with ultrasound, IFT became the essential electrotherapy disciplines ahead of all other techniques that were available in the early 1980s.

IFT continued to increase in popularity through to the 1990s, but in the early 2000s the curriculum started to change with the imposition of evidence based practice within physiotherapy and the increasing use of manual therapy.

The other issue is the use of an increasing range of drugs designed to treat a number of the conditions that physiotherapists used to treat with electrotherapy. It should be noted however, that using IFT to treat these same conditions offers an alternative for the increasing number of patients who are subject to the side effects of the drugs, or who have drug interaction problems. These conditions include low back problems, skin conditions, wounds and ulcers, certain chest conditions and even some auto-immune conditions.

Treatment with IFT, as part of a physiotherapy treatment plan, will produce better and more lasting results than medication alone. The side effects of drugs are fast becoming a serious problem with the treatment of musculo-skeletal conditions as well as with many other medical complaints. IFT has very few side effects, which are mitigated

with due training and care. There is a growing number of consultants who are actively looking for drug free therapies.

IFT is traditionally described as a low frequency current treatment that uses two medium frequency currents which "interfere" with each other to produce a beat frequency that the body recognises as a low frequency, therapeutic current.

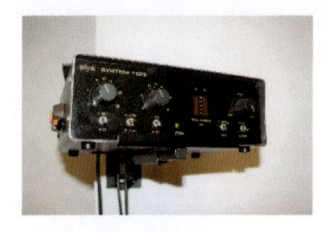

The range of this beat frequency is usually 1 - 250Hz. Although it has been established that the body can demodulate this signal, the precise mechanism is not known.

The body itself produces low frequency currents between 1 and 256Hz. These currents are produced across the cell membranes by ionic exchange, and they will vary depending on the tissue involved. By using frequencies in this range, different systems within the body can be stimulated.

ACUPUNCTURE

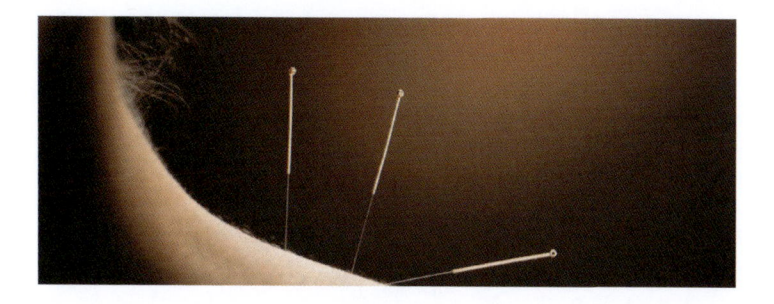

Acupuncture can be used in two ways:

Traditional acupuncture originated in China and other far eastern cultures where it is still used in mainstream healthcare, both as a stand alone therapy and in combination with conventional western medicine. Acupuncture works to help maintain the equilibrium of the body by inserting very fine needles into specific acupuncture points along pre-defined meridians on the body. This is to regulate the flow of "qi", which is the body's vital energy.
There is now a great deal of research evidence supporting acupuncture, which is gradually uncovering the mechanisms. Although it is principally known for pain relief, it does have many additional effects and benefits.

Just one area I have been exploring with acupuncture is the treatment of dysmenorrhea (painful periods), partly because low back pain is a common feature of menstruation. I have had 100% success rate so far with more than 100 patients using the two prescribed points on the legs. I don't know how it works specifically, but think it may be working via the autonomic nervous system that regulates our internal workings – to put it simply.

There is also a western version of acupuncture where we use acupuncture needles instead of injecting cortisone etc into ligaments, tendons and even joints. One effect – aside from the pain relief, is to create a small amount of micro-trauma in the injured soft tissue, which then stimulates the inflammatory process into action ie it will increase the healing rate of the injury.

It is worth noting that there are more Physiotherapists than any other healthcare profession practising acupuncture in the UK.

HEAT OR COLD?

It has passed into folk lore that in all acute conditions, cold is the treatment of choice. The theory behind this is that inflammation makes an area hot and swollen, so it would seem that cooling the area might be helpful. I do not subscribe to this opinion as I have yet to see any real evidence that cooling increases the healing rate of a condition.

Clinically, I have seen the results of people putting bags of frozen peas on ankles, backs and legs etc without realising that they are in danger of causing points of frostbite. I recently saw a patient who had pain in her buttock coming from a specific back problem and she had been advised, by a health professional, to sit on a bag of peas. She did this and caused a frostbite "burn" that covered about half of her buttock. She also still had the pain!

If you do want to apply cold, then at least do it safely ie take some ice cubes and wrap them in a damp tea towel. Then hit the pack with a rolling pin until you have crushed ice, and do not use it for more than 5 minutes.

To my mind, heat is far better and the gentle heat of wheat bags, that you heat in a microwave, is one of the most useful self help treatments on the market.

I used to work in a hospital where we saw a number of children with Still's Disease – juvenile Rheumatoid Arthritis. In this condition their joints were hot, swollen and very tender and painful. In those days, heat lamps were still just in use, but the dry heat of the lamps aggravated their joints and made them more painful. However, hydrocollator steam packs were coming onto the market and we managed to get one of these hot pack units and a cold pack unit. The steam packs worked very well for the children and the heat lamps and cold packs were a disaster! I have to say that I haven't used, or recommended any form of cold pack, for any injury, for the last 35 years or so!

There have been three of our university students on clinical placement at the clinic who could not find any significant research to support the use of ice packs ie applying cold to acute injuries. I strongly suspect that it is only used because it has been used for many years and the whole PRICE (Protection, Rest, Ice, Compression and Elevation) approach is too well entrenched now to be changed.

When I was a student, we had a clinical placement at Stoke Mandeville hospital and there we used to use ice to stimulate the bladder reflex in paraplegic patients. I would strongly suggest that you do NOT use ice packs, or frozen peas for your back pain!

I prefer my philosophy – Ice in the gin and heat on the body!

MASSAGE

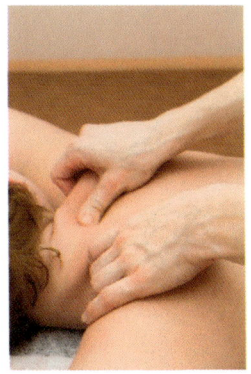

Massage used to be one of the four pillars of Physiotherapy, but is now barely taught on Physiotherapy degree courses. Manual therapy, including manipulation and mobilisations have taken over, giving us a range of techniques that are specifically targeted treatments for MSK conditions.

Over the years massage has been taken over by Sports Therapists and Sports Masseurs, straight-forward masseurs and masseuses and by any number of Beauticians and a bewildering array of different types of massage therapists.

Essentially, there are two types of massage – therapeutic/gentle massage for relaxation, and Sports massage which is more vigorous and useful after playing sport to help restore the circulation and release the tension in muscles that have been working hard during the game etc.

If you need relaxation or stress reduction, then I would suggest the more gentle approach as this can be a useful way of relieving tension from work, relationships or even families! Having treated someone with a low back problem, massage can be a useful adjunct that can sometimes help prevent further episodes.

On the other hand, sports massage is well recognised and used by sports people at almost all levels – from the top professionals to the serious amateurs.

Chapter 6

WHY IS POSTURE IMPORTANT?

Correct posture is all about mechanics (It is called biomechanics when talking about the body). Our joints are designed to work in specific ways in relation to each other, and if they are held in an abnormal position, they cannot work at their best and it can affect other joints in the whole system.

For example, try sitting or standing with your head poked forward and with rounded shoulders. Now in that position, lift your arms above your head. Note how far you can lift them. Now sit, or stand straight with your shoulders and head pulled back into a relaxed but upright position. Lift your arms above your head and note how much further you lift can now lift your arms. You should be able to reach up much further with your shoulders and neck in the better position.

If your posture is not right, then you will load all the joints in your body and create areas of stress leading to damage and pain in the human movement system.

Bad posture can also cause problems for your organs. If you round your shoulders and sit, or stand in a slumped position, then you are compressing your lungs and other organs and interfering with their ability to work at their best. Sitting and standing up tall means that your chest and lungs can fully expand. This means that you can work the lungs to their maximum capacity and get oxygen into the body to help "fuel" the whole body systems.

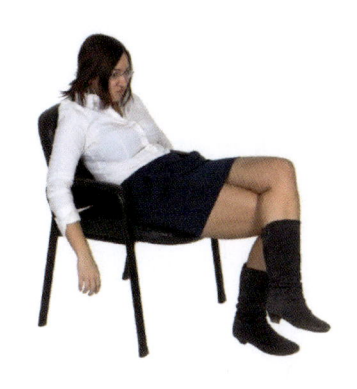

What is the best standing posture?

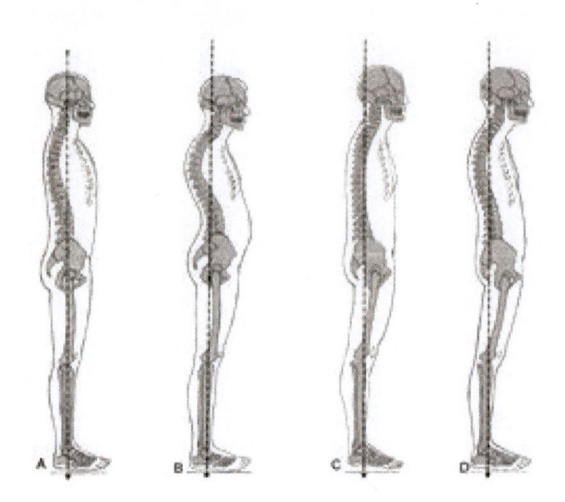

The vertical lines should pass from the ear, through the shoulder, through the side of the hip, through the centre of the knee and finally through the ankle bone.

If the weight is not correctly distributed then you will load the joints in front and behind that line.

This drawing is the correct posture and you can see what happens to the spine and other joints as the posture changes.

Posture is not just about standing up and looking good! It is really putting the body into a position that allows the skeleton and all its attachments to work in the most efficient and safe way.

Of course there are other factors that make us slump and slouch and generally look as though gravity has completely taken over, not least of which is how we feel about ourselves.

The impact on our bodies of how we feel psychologically is enormous.

If we don't like ourselves for whatever reason then it will show in our posture and the way we present ourselves to the world. Children who are taller than their peers; girls who develop larger breasts than their friends, all have issues that they cannot easily change.

To keep telling someone to stand up straight is going to have little effect unless every aspect is addressed.

Correcting the biomechanical problems of the spine and pelvis at least goes some way to dealing with the issues and can very often give the person the confidence to deal with the rest.

It is vitally important that children are encouraged to sit and stand in the right way. This will give them a positive attitude, and the best start to prevent damage to their joints and MSK systems.

Small children who sit on the floor with their legs in a W position, rather than sitting cross legged, are putting a great deal of strain on their hip joints and they should be strongly discouraged from sitting in that position.

It used to be part of the teacher's role to make the children at school sit up tall and not to slouch, but that has long since been treated as an old fashioned idea of no importance in comparison to the academic achievements, league tables and school inspector visits from OFSTED.

There is an ongoing problem with the chairs and furniture in most schools. There is only a certain amount of money allowed for school furniture and consequently most schools will go with the cheapest option.

The problem is that children do not come in standard heights.

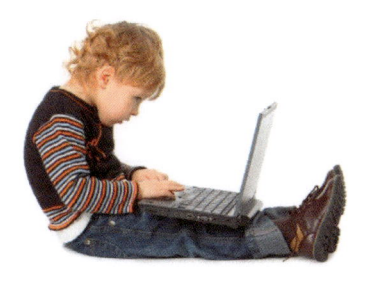

There is a huge variation in height of the children, but not in the height of desks and chairs that they are expected to sit at for many hours during the school day.

There is a great deal of time, money and effort spent on providing the right work stations for adults at work, but virtually no consideration is given to our children's workstations in school – or at home!

Another short personal story.

Some 20 years ago I carried out a small scale pilot study at my son's school. I carried out a physical assessment of 90 children, aged 9 to 11 years with a view to dividing them into 3 groups. I expected to find about 30 with minor MSK problems and 60 who had no problems. The intention was to give 2 groups of 30 children an exercise programme to improve their physical fitness and mobility and to compare them with the 3rd group of 30 who continued with the exercise programme already in place at the school.

I failed to finish the pilot because out of the 90 children, I found only 4 who had no problems at all! That was 20 years ago and the problem of the fitness of our children has only worsened to "silent" epidemic proportions. It is not just a question of diet and childhood obesity.

These problems are going to result in enormous costs to the NHS and society in general. It will cause great hardship and disability and reduce the size of the earning workforce and increase the disability costs and payments. All this is because we no longer think it is important to use our bodies in the way they were designed. Physical fitness has been relegated to a back seat for the want of an understanding of relatively simple, but vitally important problems that can be so simply resolved. How much fun did you have doing exercise and sport at school? Was it a good experience or was it a tedious part of school life that had to be endured?

The London Olympics of 2012 certainly gave a boost to sport for children, but again what of the "great grey mass" of children who are under-exercised, unfit and unwilling to take part in any physical activity for their own health? The schools are largely unable, or unwilling to stimulate children to find an activity or sport where they can succeed. Children need to understand why they need to be as fit as possible, but they also need to be shown the enjoyment that can come from feeling fit and healthy. Diet and healthy eating should be combined with exercise and sport.

In short, we are failing the vast majority of our children.

It seems to me that there is a great misunderstanding that if an answer is simple, then it cannot be worthwhile!

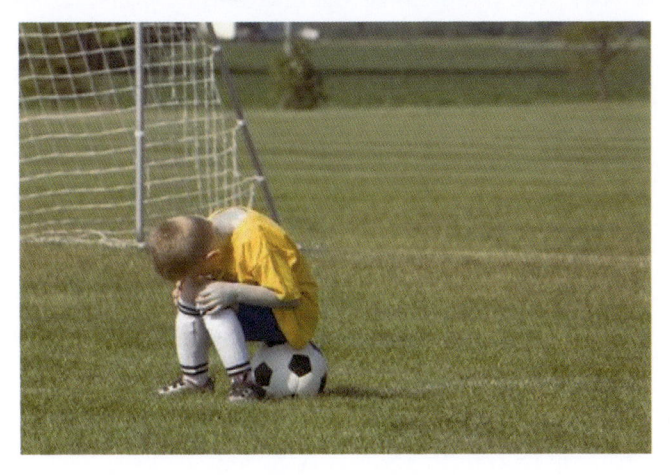

Chapter 7

MEDICATION

As a chartered physiotherapist, I cannot, nor do I wish to, prescribe drugs. That is why I trained as a physiotherapist – I have no desire to treat patients with medication/drugs or to perform surgery on them! With the required changes in the law, there are now a small number of physiotherapists who can prescribe and use drugs such as cortisone etc by injection for tendon problems for example, but again, that is not for me.

However, it is common for patients to ask my advice about what "over the counter" drugs they should consider and I will give them an outline of how certain drugs can be used for pain relief, but on the understanding that their doctor, or local pharmacist are best placed to advise them, particularly if they are on medication for other conditions. So I ask that you take the following information on the same basis.

PARACETAMOL OR IBUPROFEN?

There are a number of points that need to be considered before making a decision as to which drugs are appropriate at which point during the recovery process.

Inflammation is a normal/natural system. It is the healing process of the body. With cell activity the damaged tissue is removed and scar tissue is laid down to join soft tissue fibres like muscles and ligaments etc.

Re-modelling should then happen to reshape and restore the normal tissue again - as far as possible depending on the extent of the damage. So do you actually want to stop the body healing itself?

Ibuprofen/Nurofen belongs to a group of drugs called non steroidal anti-inflammatories (NSAID's). As the name implies, they are designed to *stop* the inflammatory process and hence the pain.

The major use of NSAIDs is for inflammatory conditions such as headaches, arthritis and back pain, but research is inconclusive as to their benefits.NSAIDs work on pain at a chemical level. They block the effects of special enzymes - specifically COX-1 and COX-2 enzymes. These enzymes play a key role in making prostaglandins, which are an essential component of the inflammatory process. By blocking these COX enzymes, NSAIDs stop your body from making as many prostaglandins. This means less swelling and less pain.

They do not act directly on the pain mechanism.

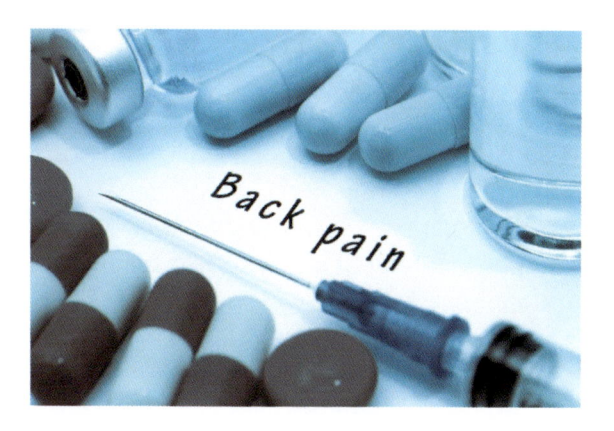

All drugs have side effects to a lesser or greater extent. NSAIDs are known to have side effects that may affect the gastro-intestinal system, and produce heart, liver and kidney problems. The longer you take them, the more likely you are to suffer from these side effects and the cost to the NHS in treating these side effects runs into millions of pounds a year.

Following a Europe-wide study, people with heart problems in the UK have been advised to stop using diclofenac, the most commonly prescribed painkiller. This advisory notice followed a 2013 Europe-wide study that confirmed at-risk patients were as much as 40% more likely to have a heart attack or stroke while taking diclofenac.

Once you stop taking the NSAID's then the inflammatory process will continue - and the pain will generally come back again. So all that has happened is that the healing process has been delayed.

A few years ago, I was at a Physiotherapy Conference on Pain and one of the keynote speakers was Nikolai Bogduk, MD, PhD. Dr. Bogduk is a professor of Pain Medicine at the University of Newcastle and the Head of the Department of Clinical Research at the Royal Newcastle Hospital in Newcastle, New South Wales, Australia.

He discussed his findings on going back to the original research on NSAIDs and reported that there was very little evidence that they had any effect at all. He also said that if he could stop doctors in Australia from prescribing the most commonly prescribed NSAID, then he could build six hospitals dedicated to musculo-skeletal medicine. I think that said it all!

Paracetamol is a simple painkiller designed to control the pain levels so that you can keep moving in a more normal way. Simple, safe and controlled movement helps stimulate the repair process.

Again, there are side effects with excessive use. If back pain is diagnosed, treated and resolved then the better it will be for everyone!

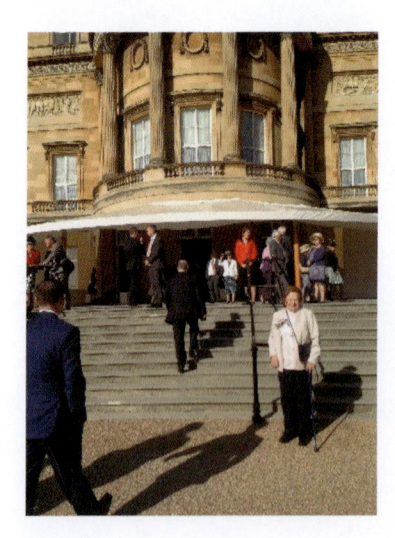

There may be a time when you need everything you can to keep the pain away and the swelling down. What if you've been invited to a Buckingham Palace Garden Party and you have just badly sprained your ankle! In this situation, you need physiotherapy treatment as soon as possible and you need both Paracetamol and Nurofen to get you through the day. You know it will delay the healing but you have to go to the Palace!

This is exactly what I said to my mother, aged 92, when she was invited to a Buckinham Palace Garden Party!

Chapter 8

NOW LET'S HAVE A SERIOUS LOOK AT ARTHRITIS

I am constantly amazed and often annoyed at how often patients are frightened by their GPs and consultants. The classic scenario is when they go to their GP complaining of back pain that started suddenly a few weeks or so before, that doesn't seem to be settling. They may be sent off for an X ray and the results come back that they have something called "lumbar spondylosis".

They are then told that they have arthritis in the back and that nothing can be done other than take pain killers and anti-inflammatories for the rest of their lives. They may be told that a "bit of physio" might help, but generally they need to try and keep moving - if they can. If it all gets too much then they may be offered an appointment with a consultant to see if there is any surgery that can be done for them.

If we look at the word "spondylosis" it comes from the Greek meaning "vertebra" and is used to mean osteoarthritis of the spine. "Lumbar spondylosis" means osteoarthritis at the bottom of the spine.

The problem here is that this is not a diagnosis, it only describes the symptoms ie pain and wear and tear in the lumbar spine. Neither is it a "death sentence" leading to a life of pain, disability and incapacity. Of course, there are the very few patients where they actually do have long term pain and disability, but the vast majority will suffer very little pain and disability more than an occasional backache after gardening, which would settle within a few days with a bit of heat and painkillers.

I have seen many X rays and scans that show really marked osteoarthritic changes, but bear little relationship to the presenting signs and symptoms. One in particular that I remember showed the last 3 vertebrae of the spine severely rotated and almost falling off each other. The scan looked as though the whole area was "rusted"! But in reality, she had hardly any pain at all in the back. A doctor looked at these scans and suggested that she should see a neurosurgeon as soon as possible. She did not do this and we treated the small amount of pain with mobilisations for the sacro-iliac joints and all was well. She was in her 70s and in all likelihood her back had been slowly getting itself into this position over many, many years. Any surgical intervention to try and straighten the spine and correct these local aberrations would do nothing except cause her long lasting pain and disability!

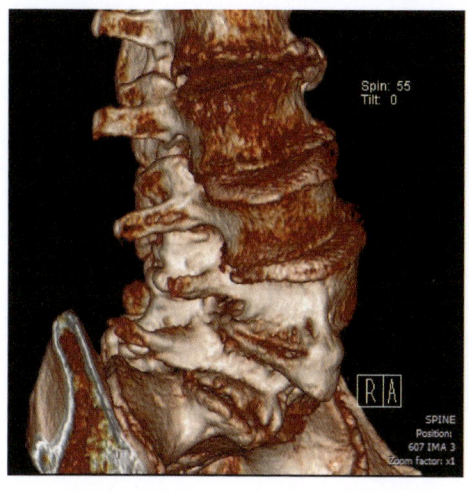

I would expect that any neurosurgeon would refuse to operate, but this hasn't always been true either in my experience. Another patient of ours, went to the doctor with pain in his back and buttock and ended up with major surgery which included putting two massive rods into the spine to fix it into a "normal" position. All this did was to nearly finish him off completely from the side effects of the surgery and medication. Bearing in mind that prior to the surgery, he was fit enough to walk up hills and the occasional mountain, it took him about 2 years to recover from the surgery - and he still had the same pain and symptoms that took him to the doctor in the first place!

So from these 2 anecdotal stories, (and my 43 years as a physiotherapist), what can I say:

Just because you can see wear and tear changes in the spine on X ray and/or scans, does not mean that osteoarthritis/lumbar spondylosis is the cause of the pain.

The body has an amazing ability to deal with problems itself. In other words, the skeleton will adapt and change according to the loading. It may well develop little outgrowths (osteophytes) that are the body's way of strutting, or fixing the problem segment to limit the movement that was causing the excessive loading. There are times when the body doesn't quite get it right and these little bony spurs can start to "grow" into the spinal nerves or even the spinal cord, but these are rare.

Just because there is narrowing of the intervertebral discs does not necessarily mean that this is what is causing your pain. Only the spaces between the vertebrae can be seen on X-ray. You cannot see the discs themselves, because they are essentially cartilage, which you cannot see on X-ray!

A good clinical examination MUST be performed before any scans or X rays. For most people, it is the clinical examination that will provide the answers. It is the clinical examination that will indicate any serious pathology that needs a scan and/or X ray to confirm the problem or the severity of the problem.

For example, a clinical examination can indicate a problem with an intervertebral disc. It will also give a very good indication of the severity of that lesion by identifying degrees of nerve involvement or damage, but there are also the Red Flags that say that this patient has a more severe problem that may well need surgery. This situation definitely needs all the necessary scans etc to confirm the diagnosis.

Scans and X rays should not be considered the first line in the diagnostic process as they can throw up all sorts of red herrings and blind alleys. These cost far more than a good clinician carrying out a detailed clinical examination. It is the way of medicine these days that has led us to think that we have to be able to "see" the problem before making a diagnosis and that somehow, carrying out a detailed system of checks and tests and balances founded in sound anatomy, biomechanics and neuro-orthopaedics, tried and tested over many years, is somehow inferior to someone interpreting what they think they can see on an MRI - or even worse, ignoring the patient reporting a set of symptoms that bear no relationship what ever to what is seen on the scans.

Lumbar spondylosis does not happen suddenly. The changes happen slowly over many years. So the first question has to be, "How did the problem come on?" If you got sudden low back pain bending over to pick up something off the floor, then it cannot be coming from spondylosis - regardless of what the X rays and scans show. This equally applies to back pain that comes on over a couple of days.

Lumbar spondylosis? So what! Providing there is no associated nerve damage or unremitting severe pain, or other Red Flag signs, then I would be looking elsewhere for the cause of the symptoms.

Chapter 9

FEAR AND ANXIETY

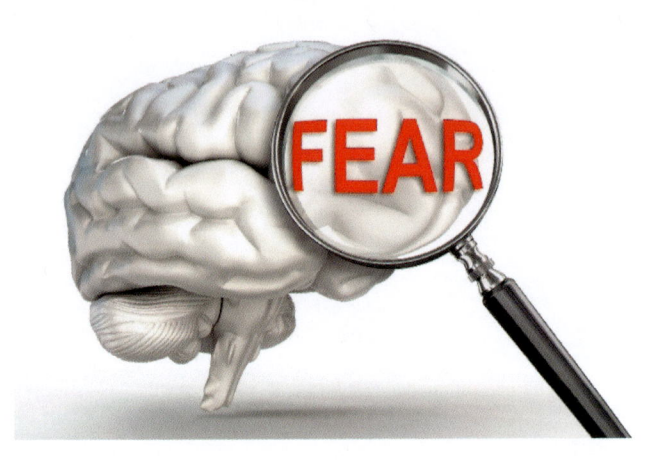

If we can take away people's fears about their condition, then we are half way to making them better. This takes education, understanding and one to one contact for as long as is necessary.

The interpersonal skills needed for a successful outcome are arguably the top of the list when providing a health service, but this aspect is fast taking a back seat in the face of budgets and cost cutting.

It is also extremely difficult to research and evaluate as an essential component of "best practice", because we are talking about human care and skills that are not measurable in terms of doses, or so many "pills taken only with food".

What is being missed is that dealing with people's fears well, is the most cost effective approach. "Take the fear" and further pain and complications will be markedly reduced giving a saving to the healthcare costs and people's ongoing disability and misery. The only cost here is time. There are no drug or medication costs.

Physiotherapists spend more time with patients -when they are awake, than any other healthcare profession and are ideally placed, with the skills and the knowledge, to provide this all important service. Historically this is what we were trained to do. To get the best results, you have to have a partnership between the patient and the physiotherapist. It has to be teamwork, but this relationship is being eroded in the NHS by cutting the appointment times and therefore increasing the waiting lists. If it carries on in this way then the future of NHS physiotherapy will come under question and the patients will suffer even more.

Dealing with patients' fears is an area that I find is getting to be more and more of an issue. It seems to be a rapidly growing problem: tests, procedures and even surgery are being carried out with little explanation to the patients themselves and virtually no follow up to explain the findings or help with the rehabilitation process. I am only talking about back pain and the myriad of other musculo-skeletal conditions as this is my experience. I do not presume to make this a universal comment.

This lack of information and discussion is generating fear in people who have been through all sorts of pain and disability, which in turn is making the pain and disability worse. They don't know when or how to move, to go back to work or simply how to resume their normal life.

In the days when there were enough physiotherapists and other medical staff in the hospitals, then patients had access to all the services they needed within a reasonable time frame. Now it seems that the majority are sent away with nothing but a sheet of generic exercises and possibly a follow up appointment 6 weeks later. What is it about our health care system that everything revolves around 6 weeks? Is it a significant historical or mathematical number that has been shown to influence the outcome of medical procedures? Or is it that everything should be getting better within that month and a half, so there will be less to do if you leave the patient that long on their own?!

Maybe I am being too cynical, but I think this is getting to be a serious problem of lack of communication.

The other problem now is that it seems that it has become an accepted fact that out patient physiotherapy appointments in the NHS are even more difficult to get than an appointment with the GP. It is not uncommon for physiotherapy waiting lists to be many months. What this means is that every patient that eventually gets their physiotherapy appointment has become a chronic pain patient with all the extra problems that chronic pain can bring. This of course assumes that the patient hasn't gone elsewhere, such as the independent sector, because they couldn't wait any longer to find the answer to their problems.

What seems to be the issue here is that medical people can have the tendency to forget that the patient in front of them has little or no knowledge of the workings of their bodies. Spending time talking to our patients would very quickly show the limit of their knowledge. Why should they know very much unless they had also spent years at university learning all the anatomy and pathology? They may know a great deal about their own work, but nothing about how their bodies work or could go wrong.

I have met many patients who are really terrified to move. They are frightened that if they move in the wrong way then their back may fall apart in some way, or that the discs may completely rupture and they will then become paralysed. They have simply not been told what they can or cannot do to make things better. No-one explained exactly what was wrong in terms that they could understand. No-one thought to teach them what they can or cannot do and why? This is what rehabilitation is all about. These days "rehabilitation" is the latest buzz word, bandied about as if it has only just been thought of! There are many different healthcare people apparently providing it, but there is precious little evidence that rehabilitation is actually being provided for the patients. In reality, it is what most of the Physiotherapy profession is all about. It is what we have been providing for the last 115 years. It is where the profession started.

Physiotherapists are in fact the experts in this area, but the current delivery of the service is being cut back so much that they cannot provide this very necessary service in the 20 minutes they are allowed to treat the patients. This is why there are other healthcare professionals and even personal fitness trainers offering some sort of service in the name of rehabilitation. The general public are being denied the essential aftercare, so they are looking elsewhere, and other people are picking up the slack in the system.

It is not a costly exercise, unlike prescribing drugs, to provide patients with enough information about their condition and how to deal with it.

What can you do if you have something wrong that you don't understand, or are worried about your future with this problem?

Ask whoever you are seeing what they think is the full diagnosis. If they can't tell you then go to someone who can. This may mean a referral from your GP. What you need is a second opinion. Make sure that they give you enough time to fully explain everything in terms that you can understand. Make sure that all your fears are dealt with.

Then you will be in a position to move forward and work towards getting better.

Make sure that whoever you go to, that they have genuine, recognised qualifications. Do not assume that just because they have some letters after their name, that they are qualified to treat you. Check on the internet what the letters after the name stand for and whether there is a regulatory body. Check that there is Professional Indemnity cover for the members of the regulatory and/or Professional Body. Professional Indemnity is insurance in case anything goes wrong. It is only available for health professionals who have recognised qualifications.

There is a world of difference in knowledge, skills and ability between someone who completes a 6 week course at a local further education college and someone who has completed a 4000 hour honours degree course at university and then spent years in a clinical setting and completing many hours of post graduate education and courses, who is also regulated under a government established regulatory body as well as their governing professional body!

Chapter 10

PAIN

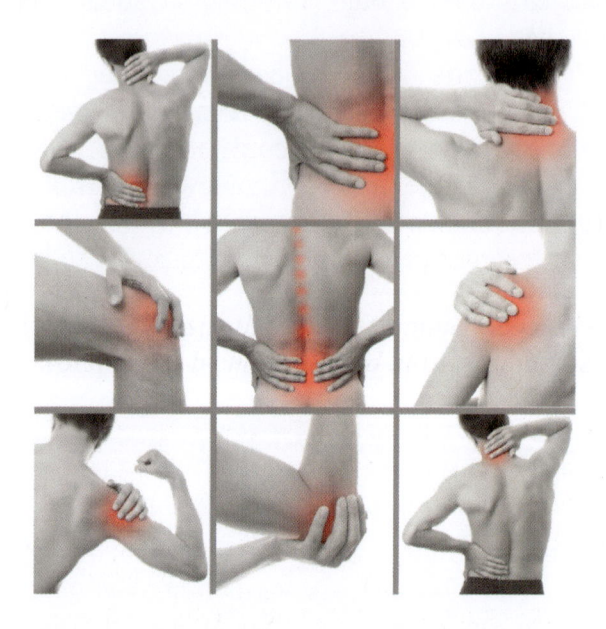

"No pain, no gain" & *"Pain equals harm"*

How many people still believe these phrases to be true? I would estimate that most people still think they are true.

We now know far more about how the pain mechanism works and I will try and give you a very simplified version. I have put into the footnotes just some of the books that you might find interesting to read if you would like to know more.

A LITTLE HISTORY OF PAIN

Since the "medical dawn of time", people have thought that if you stand on something sharp, then a message goes up to your brain to say that you are injured and a corresponding message comes down from the brain, to the required muscles, to make you take your foot off the sharp object. Seems sensible! The brain is trying to protect you from hurting yourself even more, so it makes you do things that will stop you causing even more problems.

But what about pain that carries on, unrelenting, for years? What about those people who apparently don't feel pain when they are obviously injured and yet manage to walk away from accidents etc?

Pain clinics were set up in the 1940s in an attempt to help patients with ongoing, or "chronic pain". The medical view was that these patients had psychological problems and were therefore put under the care of the psychiatrists. In some way, they thought, these patients were either suffering from hysterical pain, or they were lying for some reason.

It was not until 1965 that the Gate Control Theory of Pain was put forward by Professors Ron Melzack and Patrick Wall that ideas and treatment protocols began to change.[2]

Essentially what they proposed was that there was a physiological gate in the spinal cord that could be shut to stop pain messages going up to the brain - in effect analgaesia. This happens because chemicals could be produced, by the body, that would block the transmission of the nerve impulses up to the brain.

This can happen when we are distracted from the pain. Your child falls over and hurts his knee. You pick him up, rub the knee and maybe give him a sweet. His brain has become more interested in the unexpected sweet and effectively stops thinking about the injury to his knee. As adults, we also do this by burying our heads in work, or a hobby, to literally "take our minds off" the fact that we have a pain in the foot when we sprained an ankle last week! What has happened is that the "gate has been shut."

Since this ground breaking work was done in the 60s, there has been a great deal of research and studies, that have given us an even greater understanding of the complexities of the pain mechanisms. Particular physiotherapists around the world have played a major role in expanding our knowledge and developing

---

[2] **The Challenge of Pain** Ronald Melzack and Patrick D Wall ISBN 978-0-140-25670-3

new ways to help patients in pain, whether this is acute, or chronic pain.

Notably:

Louis Gifford FCSP[3] British physiotherapist
David Butler[4] Australian
David Butler and Lorimer Moseley[5] Australian

CURRENT PAIN CONCEPTS

We are born with a brand new brain and nervous system. All the parts are there and the nervous system is like a new computer. It has the operating system already installed, but you have yet to put any software on it.

In effect, think of the brain as the central processing unit (CPU). As you learn to use the computer, you will add software and change its settings, screensaver and display. In effect you want to personalise it!

As you use it to do different things, like write books, then the document will be saved on the hard drive. This means you can access the book later and maybe do some more work on it!

The brain works in a similar way to the CPU. The CPU is constantly monitoring the whole system to make sure all its components are working at their best, and any problems will bring up an error message, like "Printer off line" or the 404 error message when you try and access a website online!

If you think about it, the brain is constantly monitoring all our systems and internal workings to make sure that we are not too hot or cold; that the heart and lungs are responding to what we are actively doing like running the odd marathon; that all the glands are producing what they should and in the right amounts or that the liver and kidneys are doing their job properly depending on what we put down our throats!

All of these activities, and infinitely more, are happily going along doing their thing under the control of the brain and

---

[3] **Aches and Pains** Louis Gifford CNS Press 9-70953-342358
[4] **The Sensitive Nervous System** David Butler
[5] **Explain Pain**

we are usually totally unaware of all these processes. To do this though, the brain has to have a constant feedback system from all our component parts telling it what is going on. Equally, there has to be a system that can modify the behaviour of all these systems to take into account what we, as individuals, are doing at that moment.

It may be that we need to modify our **conscious** behaviour to keep these **subconscious** processes carrying on in the best way. For example, we learn that to go out in the snow with very little clothes on, could drop our body temperature to a dangerous level and the body systems need to have a pretty constant temperature to work. So the brain sends out messages to both the body (shivering) and to other parts of the brain, to say that you are being stupid here, go and put some clothes on!

As we grow up, we learn what is good for us and what is not so good. These learning experiences effectively rewrite the software of our brains.

We know that very painful experiences, especially in childhood, can make the nervous system very sensitive. We also know that people whose parents were over cautious and excessively protective, can make them actually feel more pain in their adult lives, to the same apparent injury suffered by others. Parents who say to their children, "Come on, it is only a minor scratch. Get back on your bike and you will be fine" are actually helping their child's nervous system to be able to damp down pain messages when it is needed. Of course I am not saying that if the child has actually broken his leg, that he should be told to "Man up"!! But, constructive help to get him through a painful, difficult time really does have physiological benefits for him in the future.

This is where pain gating comes in. This is the ability of the brain and nervous system to decide when a situation is dangerous to the whole body and when it is necessary to **stop** the pain from a minor injury in order to avoid possible serious injury, or even death. Simply, we have the ability to decide whether we want, or need, to feel pain depending on the situation. This can be a physical, or psychological situation.

VERY IMPORTANT POINT:

Pain is real
It cannot be manufactured
It can be moderated

We now understand the mechanisms where stress, physical or mental, can severely impact on the ability of the brain and nervous system to control pain. Although this seems an obvious thing to say, we now understand the mechanisms and the effects on the body.

Pain can be shut down by "closing the gate", but we also know that it can be made worse, and even persistent and continuous, by "holding that gate open". This is chronic pain.

In Louis Gifford's terms, pain can be "bottom up" where there is actual tissue damage causing the pain messages to be recognised by the brain as a possible danger to the body, or it can be "top down" where the gate is still wide open in spite of the fact that the tissue damage was repaired long ago.

How does this happen?

In its very simplest form, the software of the nervous system has been re-programmed.

You may have bent over to pick something up from the floor. You felt something "go" in your back and you suffered the most intense pain that you had ever felt. This event re-programmes your software to associate bending over with intense pain. So in order to stop you damaging your back again in the future, your brain will open the "pain gate" every time you start to bend over. What has happened is that low level sensations like stretching, which the brain would normally "ignore", become much more intense i.e. painful.

This doesn't happen with everyone. There has to be something else in the software that has triggered the sensitivity to a level of "red alert". The problem still remains that you are feeling pain, and "traditional conditioning" is telling you that there must be something wrong with your body.

And of course everyone who is trying to help you get rid of the pain, who doesn't appreciate what is going on here, will try every trick in the book to try and find the problem tissue that they also think is causing the pain.

It is still a common approach to apply every scan, blood test and medical examination in the book to find the source, to a point where the chronic pain patient finds themselves on a medical treadmill that may well end up with increased medication, or even surgically burning off the nerve endings in the spine in the vain hope that this will stop the pain.

The fact is that the pain is generated by the nervous system and is being influenced and enhanced by almost every system in the brain and body. Every experience you have ever had; everything you have seen – even on television or films; every conversation you have had; every injury; every simple ache and pain goes together to make up You, as a unique individual.

You experience pain in a way that is Your Way and it is going to be different from everyone else. It has nothing to do with so called "Pain thresholds". It is absolutely the way that Your nervous system works. It is vitally important that you understand that pain is the result of Your nervous system deciding that now is a good time for you to feel pain in order for you as an individual can survive.

Simply treating tissues and tissue injury is not going to relieve the pain until Your nervous system has decided that You no longer need to feel pain. In Louis Gifford's terms - Treating from the "bottom up" is never going to work on it's own. It needs an approach that is "top down". In other words, you can provide the best treatment in the world that research has shown will cure and resolve a condition, but if Your nervous system and You, as an individual person, given all Your experiences continues to think that You are under threat – then you will feel pain.

How can this pain be treated then if the pain is not coming from damaged tissue?

If you are in this situation, then you need to find someone who has the knowledge and understanding of how to help you manage and even eliminate the pain. It is outside the remit of this book to go into the detail of just how this can be done. However there are a number of studies and research that has been done to help you understand that this is a problem NOT in your mind, but is a definite, and real condition that can be helped, and even cured.

There are a number of instances I have read about that really support the research and concepts:

There are people who suffer phantom limb pain in a limb that they never had as a congenital defect. The point here is that the cells in the brain and nerves in the spinal cord are there that would have gone into the limb if they had it. So the pain has to be generated centrally as it cannot possibly be coming from damaged cells in the absent limb. Fascinating!

From Louis Gifford's book Aches and Pains - In the 1950s, a study was done looking at a surgical procedure in the 1930s by a surgeon named Feischi. He thought that by tying off small blood vessels (the internal mammary arteries) in the chest, above the heart, that the circulation would be improved to the heart in cases of angina pectoralis. This operation appeared to work, but no-one could find out why. When some of these patients died and post mortem examinations were carried out, there was no sign of the suggested increase in the circulation to the heart. But the patients concerned had far less problems with the angina after the surgery.

The study in the 1950s, repeated the operation on some patients, but did a sham operation on others ie they went through an "operation" and had a scar to prove it, but none of the arteries were tied off. Interestingly, the patients who had the sham operation got better, and their ECGs improved!

So what was going on there?

To put it very simply, it was the placebo effect. The brain was convinced that it was going to work and the body healed itself!

The body has an enormous capacity to heal itself if we know how to tap into the process, but is surgery the way to tap into it? There are obviously times when surgery is really needed to puts "bits" back together, or cut out "bits" that we shouldn't have, but I would suggest that you think very hard about these quotes if surgery is offered to you for your chronic pain problem:

'Surgery has the most potent placebo effect that can be exercised in medicine' and *'The history of medicine is the history of the placebo'!*

Do you want to go through a surgical procedure, that in itself is a trauma to the body and your nervous system, when there are non surgical (and non medication) techniques available that will equip you with the ability to control and even remove your pain?

The Mature Organism Model proposed by Louis Gifford is probably the most significant milestone in our understanding of pain since the Pain Gate Theory put forward by Melzack and Wall in the 1960s. For those of you who want to know more detail of these concepts, then I would suggest that you Google the names or the theories.

This is my very simplified version of a very complex mechanism. It is how I try an explain it to my patients:

Your brain and nervous system is working hard to protect you – as an entire person - from harm. If there is damage to some part of it, be it disease or injury, then the tissues involved send signals to the brain to say that they are damaged and stressed.

The brain meanwhile, is constantly monitoring how the whole body is doing from an entire system of feedback from all the components of the body. It will pick up the signals from the damaged tissues and then decide what to do about it. This decision is made by accessing all the stored information that it has from every experience you have ever had. It also takes into account the immediate environment and whether there is a greater threat from outside the body.

If there is, then the brain and nervous system will take action to get you out of even more harms way. It is a decision as to whether there is more danger coming from outside than inside. In other words, is it better to stay where you are, or to move to a place of safety where the body and brain can then turn "inwards" to deal with the problems inside? It is why we take ourselves to bed when we are feeling unwell. Our bed is a place of safety, and sleep in a safe environment allows the brain to mobilise the "night shift" (as Louis describes!) to come on and start to repair any injury or damage.

This is why people feel pain AFTER an accident and not necessarily at the time of the injury. As an aside, it is also why people may be involved in a car accident and not really be aware of any injury until some while later, and that plays havoc for the medical profession in trying to decide whether this person has a genuine whiplash injury from the accident! If the health professional doesn't have the necessary MSK skills and knowledge of pain mechanisms, then they will miss the genuine case as well as the "insurance opportunist".

Once you understand this mechanism, then you can appreciate why we feel pain. It is the brain that decides whether there will be pain and not the tissues under threat. The amount of pain we feel is also a decision made by the brain that has accessed **all** our experiences and associated emotions. It is also why we may feel pain long after the original injury is healed ie Chronic Pain. In this situation the brain and nervous system continues to create pain because it has learnt from experience that certain movements or actions caused problems in the past and again it is trying to protect you from futher harm.

Chronic pain needs a completely different approach, because now the treatment has to be directed to the brain and nervous system – and very much, the person behind the brain. I like to think of it as re-programming the software of the nervous system that has developed a "bug" in its system. What needs to happen here is for the patient themselves to understand the mechanism and to realise that the pain they are feeling is NOT a threat to them, or their tissues. In other words – pain does not equal harm!

This is a relatively new area of work for we health professionals and is far more complex than I have laid it out here.

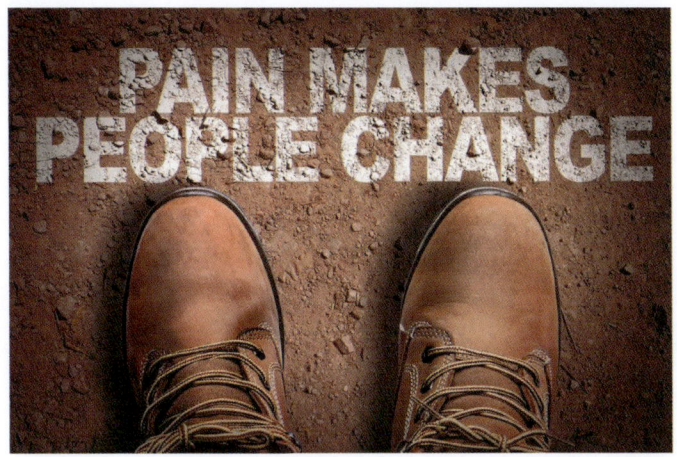

It often needs a multi-disciplinary approach and medication is only a small part of the whole. The key point I would like to say is that if MSK problems are treated correctly and efficiently in the very early stages then chronic pain would not develop. It is by feeding people's fears and worries in these important early stages, that chronic pain develops. Brushing off a patient's very real fears and worries as making a fuss etc will only make matters worse, feed the fears and make the whole problem worse.

To close this section, I would like to re-state my original thought:

My job is to stop acute problems becoming chronic ones.

FOR PEOPLE WITH ACUTE OR SUB ACUTE PAIN
Louis Gifford FCSP

Some years ago, Louis allowed me to reproduce this list of Do's and Do nots for people in pain for our Back Book that we use in the clinic. I have reproduced it here as it still holds true and is supported by all the work that he did in his clinical professional life, in order to help the millions of people who suffer on a daily basis.

This list is not just for people with back pain, but it applies to everyone with acute and sub acute pain. Thank you Louis once again.

TRYING TO CREATE THE CONDITIONS NEEDED FOR THE BEST CHANCES OF TISSUE RECOVERY and RETURN TO HEALTH

Some practical guidelines which are based on current, well researched literature, into the prevention of chronic (ongoing) low back pain conditions.

- ✓ Try and avoid highly stressful situations, feelings of anxiety, anger, frustration about the problem.
- ✓ Even though it may be difficult, it is best to accept and adjust to what has happened. Try and alter other parts of your life that are also a source of anxiety or tension. This can be extremely helpful.
- ✓ The reason for this is that "stress/feeling uptight/anxious" tends to dampen down the body's natural healing mechanisms.
- ✓ Reduce mental and physical pressures on yourself as much as possible.
- ✓ Calmness and acceptance; positive attitude to recovery.
- ✓ Good sleep, good diet.
- ✓ It is helpful to avoid/cut down on toxins-alcohol, smoking, unhealthy environments.
- ✓ Avoid prolonged inactivity, excessive rest (lying and sitting especially).

- ✓ Intersperse short periods of rest with gentle and progressively more activity.
- ✓ Your physiotherapists will give you clear guidelines about what to do and how to do it.
- ✓ Try and make resting "time dependent" and not "pain dependent".
- ✓ Being guided by the pain often leads to long rests after big increases in pain. It is not a good idea to keep going until the pain comes on.
- ✓ Keep the activity to a level that won't cause long-lasting pain.
- ✓ High levels of ongoing pain are not only frustrating, but also lead you into what is called the under-activity-over activity cycle.
- ✓ Continuous over-activity, with a consequent increase, or flare up, in the pain for many hours or even days leads to a far less overall activity with a consequent reduction in tissue and general health.
- ✓ Regular short rests of the tissues, even when the pain is not particularly bad, is the best way to use rest. For example, 5 minutes every hour in the very early stages.
- ✓ Perform gentle exercises after resting and before moving. This prepares the body and painful area for movement.
- ✓ Progressive stretching and strengthening exercises are an important part of recovery. Your physiotherapist will teach you and advise you.
- ✓ You may have found your own movements that feel good and loosen you up. Use them!
- ✓ Try to avoid overdoing any one thing, and not varying your activities.
- ✓ Early after the injury, take care not to over-exert the injured part with excessive, sudden forces.
- ✓ Even here there is unlikely to be increased damage, but quite likely to be an increase in pain.
- ✓ The key is to increase the loading and the speed of loading, in a gradual and controlled manner.
- ✓ The tissues have to slowly rebuild their fitness and tolerance of the things that cause discomfort.

- ✓ Introducing exercises that have a speed and more sudden element to them will be introduced into your programme at an appropriate point.
- ✓ Regular movements of the injured tissues and getting back normal movement in a progressive and well controlled way is important.
- ✓ Maintain confidence in the strength of the tissues.
- ✓ Always discuss any worries you have with your physiotherapist.
- ✓ Being anxious about the pain or about damage, prevents your return of confidence in the painful part.
- ✓ Get any worries sorted!
- ✓ Maintaining adequate exercise for the rest of the body.
- ✓ Plenty of light ie time out of doors-feeling good and continuing to enjoy life helps a great deal.
- ✓ Keep socialising!!
- ✓ Adherence to exercises and advice.
- ✓ If you cannot see the point of the exercises, or the activities suggested, or cannot fit them into your life, then tell your physiotherapists. They will discuss or redesign the programme for you. This is vital.
- ✓ Staying mentally occupied-early return to work/normal activities is highly desirable. If this is not possible, then keep occupied with hobbies or other activities.
- ✓ Sitting at home doing nothing, waiting for the pain to go away or a cure to be found has been shown to be unhelpful.
- ✓ Try not to become preoccupied by the pain or the injured part. Giving pain a great deal of attention helps to make its presence a habit.
- ✓ Try not to pin all your hopes on any one clinician to cure you.
- ✓ Being totally passive (meaning inactive in the recovery process, and relying on the therapist to cure you) is missing a very large percent of the recovery potential.
- ✓ The best clinicians provide guidance and help, show you how to improve the local tissue conditions and

chances for recovery, but very rarely provide a whole cure.
- ✓ Patients are urged to understand that they have a major role to play in their recovery and health eg in diabetes, insulin tablets or injections alone are not enough to ensure health.
- ✓ If with diabetes, one eats cream cakes every afternoon, take little exercise, and insist on drinking a bottle of wine with dinner, the illness will soon be out of control.
- ✓ Insulin alone does not ensure health. Some thoughtful reconstruction of one's daily habits is also required.
- ✓ Heart surgery helps a desperately sick heart, but it has been shown that even here, lifestyle changes can reverse this damage to the extent that many patients can actually avoid having surgery.
- ✓ Lifestyle changes here included gentle regular exercise, good diet, the use of relaxation techniques and the use of mental reasoning techniques that help to reduce unhelpful emotions such as fear and anxiety that are generated in stressful situations.
- ✓ Discuss and ask questions. If you have any worries or misgivings about anything, it is important that they are convincingly dealt with.
- ✓ Conflicting information is especially unhelpful-it must be sorted out.
- ✓ Make sure you fully understand the nature of your condition, the potential for recovery and the strength of the tissues involved.
- ✓ There is nothing worse than having a constant fear of re-damaging a structure or exacerbating high levels of pain.
- ✓ Discuss the use and value of painkilling drugs with your physiotherapist.
- ✓ Make sure you have been given strategies to help you control your pain.

Examples here are: relaxation techniques (simple breathing exercises), regular short rests interspersed with activity, exercises that feel good, heat, ice/cold, and in some cases, the use of TENS can be a help.

Medication may be vital for the control of very high levels of pain in the early stages. It has been clearly shown that when high levels of pain at the onset of a problem are well controlled the problem resolves far quicker and the patient returns to normal function and work sooner.

Discuss any worries you have about tablets and their side effects with your doctor or physiotherapist.

Whatever your age, healing and recovery are still very much a possibility-it is true that healing and recovery are slower as we get older. We are also likely to have some wear and tear changes in our muscles, ligaments and joints.

This is quite normal and is not necessarily painful. Gradual improvement of fitness and function in a way that you feel comfortable with and have no worries about, encourages faster recovery, will lead to a far better state of health and also to lowered levels of pain.

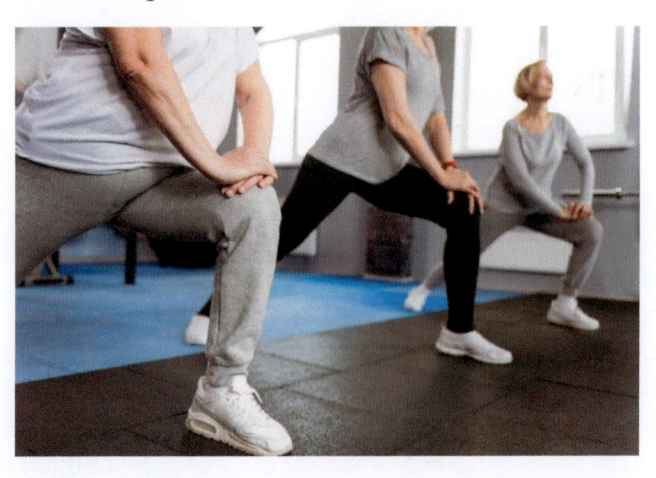

Anyone can get fitter at any age

Anyone can recover from an injury at any age

For some it is easier than others

Chapter 11

DOS & DON'TS OF BACK CARE

Don't put your head down when bending forward

This loads 2/3 of your body weight onto the last joints of the spine - before you put anything in your hands.

Keep your nose up and your bottom out when bending forward.

The half bend position is the worst for backs, such as cleaning your teeth! LEAN on the basin or the wall.

If you need to bend forward then lean on something to take the strain off your back.

If you have to bend down to load the washing machine or the dishwasher, lean on the machine, or your knees.
If you want to bend forward when you are gardening, lean on your knees with your elbows, or get onto all fours keeping one hand on the ground.
Do keep the small hollow in your back. So if you are sitting put a small cushion/rolled up towel in your back-even in your car!

Don't do the same activity for more than half an hour at a time.

The body doesn't like being in the same position for lengthy periods of time. Our bodies have joints and muscles and things to allow us to move The old adage "if you don't use it - you lose it" still holds true! Keep changing the activity.

Use a kitchen timer and set it for 30mins - whatever you are doing and including sitting at work in front of a computer. When the 30mins is up, just change your position. Do a few stretches. Walk around the chair if that is all you can manage. It only needs a few minutes to allow the body to re-adjust and get itself ready for the next 30 minutes. Fidgeting in your chair is the order of the day. Concentration levels are better for having a short break as well!

Do keep your shoulders relaxed when sitting at the computer

So often, we sit at the computer and after a while - if we realise, our shoulders have risen up almost to our ears. This will certainly happen when we are lost in our work and concentrating. But this will set up tension in the upper trapezius muscles and can cause headaches as well as neck pain. So consciously make the effort to drop your shoulders and relax the muscles on either side.

Try and sit upright at your computer

Try putting one leg tucked underneath the chair to keep the hollow in the low back.
If you sit on the edge of the chair, put one foot tucked underneath the chair with the other foot on the flat on the floor, then you will find that you automatically sit up in the right position.
Research shows that the only time we use the back of a chair is when we lean back to relax in between bursts of activity.
If we need to answer the phone etc when sitting at the computer, then we are even less likely to use the back rest on the chair. However good the chair, there are few occasions when workers actually sit in a chair as shown on the box! Providing the chair, desk, keyboard and screen are at the right relative heights, then you should have no problems.
If you sit correctly, then your body will support itself and expensive chairs are unnecessary.
Do keep your wrists off the desk Allow the free movement of the hands at the keyboard.

Laptop computers should not be used on your lap – despite the name!

Laptops should be used for short bursts of computer work and they are not intended for putting on your lap, slumped on a settee, or on a coffee table.
If you habitually use a laptop on a desk at work, then get a PC. That way you can get the workstation setup right for you to spend the hours necessary without strain on the body.
There are any number of accessories that you can get to effectively turn laptops into PCs. It must surely be cheaper to buy a PC in the first place!

If you have a computer at home, set it up as if you were in an office

The same rules apply. Children and adults alike!

Don't sit slumped in the armchair in the evenings

That only puts extra bending strain on the spine at all levels. You don't have to sit bolt upright - that puts even more loading down the spine. Put a small cushion in the small of your back and sit back at about 120° with your head and neck supported.
If you look at old wing type chairs, the people that made them knew what was comfortable! Unfortunately, the modern design of chair and settee has short backs and long seats, so few people can actually sit correctly and comfortably without causing strain on their spine.

Don't sleep on the floor, or a bed that is too firm

You need a bed/mattress that supports your body and yet allows the bony bits of you to sink into the mattress.
In other words, your shoulders and hips need to be able to sink into the bed allowing the spine to take up a neutral position. In this way, the spinal joints and muscles can relax and recover from the stresses of the day.

Don't sleep with more than one pillow

If you need to have your head higher for other reasons eg chest problems, then raise the head end of the bed on house bricks or wooden blocks.

The pillow doesn't have to be skinny, and you can have 2 very thin pillows if you prefer. The important point is that there should be enough thickness of pillow to fill out the bit between your ear and shoulder when you are lying on your side.

If you have a thicker pillow, then when you lie on your back, it will push your head forward - the same as when you are sitting and poking your chin forward. This puts strain onto the small joints on the side of the neck and loads the rest of the spine as a result.

Do adjust the driving position to 130 degrees

The best driving position is not sitting bolt upright, but as with sitting in the evening, you should incline the seat, and even put a small cushion/rolled up towel in the hollow of your back.

KEEP MOVING! that's what the body is designed to do!

Staying in one position means that you will get set and stiffen up. So keep pottering about.
When you first wake up, bend up your knees and roll them from side to side for a few minutes until your back has loosened up a little.

SOME THINGS YOU MAY NOT HAVE THOUGHT ABOUT!

Situps, and stomach crunches, are really not good for you.

They are good for our business, as Physiotherapists, but not for you!
Think of it this way - lying on the floor with your knees bent, and then coming up into a sit-up, or crunch position is exactly the same movement as sitting on a chair and brings both knees up to your chest. One exercise is carried out with you horizontal, and

the other you are vertical. The thing is that it uses the same muscles. These are the muscles that bend your hips! There is some work from the abdominals, but actually very little!

Sit-ups and crunches really load the low back because you are going to round the back, and flatten out the lumbar curve. These exercises will not give you a six pack – they will give you strong hip flexors! They may work the abdominals a little, but not enough!

The McGill curl up is the best exercise for getting good abdominals and I have included it in the Exercise section of this book. If you go to YouTube and look for "Waterloo's Dr. Spine, Stuart McGill". He has an excellent video talking about the myths of back pain and the right exercises to do.

Roll on your side getting out of bed

Following on from No Sit-ups – when you get up from lying, don't come straight up, because you are again loading the spine. Instead, roll over on to one side and sit up sideways from there – pushing yourself up with your hands. This puts the least amount of strain on your low back.

I would suggest that you always get up like this from lying – even if you don't have back pain.

Put your "headlights on full beam". In other words – lift your chest

This comes under the POSTURE heading. What you need to think is that your chest, male or female, has headlights on the front! You want to make sure that these headlights are on Full Beam and not Dipped, whether you are sitting, or standing, or walking.

Sit with knee tucked under the chair

This is one for anyone who spends time at a computer – meaning anything from an hour to a full working day, and at work, or at home.

Sit on the edge of the chair with one foot flat on the floor. Now tuck the other foot underneath the chair. What you should find has just happened is that the pelvis has rocked forward and you now have a small curve in the hollow of your back. In this position, your spine should be able to take the load of sitting, and it should feel quite comfortable and effortless to sit there at your desk.

If you "jiggle" the knee with the foot tucked under you, then you are gently rocking the pelvis and keeping movement going in the low back. This position is very similar to the Kneeling Stools that were popular some years ago, but which fell out of fashion because it is difficult, from a cultural point of view, to sit on a stool at work – particularly if you happen to be a Chief Executive!!!

Equally, wriggle in your seat every so often. It may annoy the people around you, but you are keeping the flexibility and muscle activity going, which in turn will reduce the likelihood of low back pain. It is also useful if you have low back pain, so it is part of treatment/management as well as prevention.

Loading and unloading the car

You go shopping to the supermarket. You have bought enough food for the week and it comes in half a dozen or so plastic bags. What natural law is in action where you can fill a trolley as you shop, but it wont' fit in the trolley after you pack it into bags? Why is it that there is no room for the 9 pack of toilet rolls anymore?

Anyway. Here you are, struggling to the car trying to manage the trolley with a faulty wheel with the toilet rolls under your arm. You get to your car and then have to find the keys. This you manage and you open the boot.

Your car is a nice hatchback and you had prepared the car for all the shopping by putting down the back seats. Now you start to unload the trolley. Sensibly you think that you should empty the first of the bags furthest into the car, but that's a bit of a stretch and you commit the cardinal error of bending forward, unsupported, and with an extra weight in your hands. It is no wonder that you suffer sudden low back pain!

To avoid this situation, very simply think about how you are going to load the car. If your can, put one knee into the car so that you shorten the lever on your back and you can control the movement. The other major point here is to keep your head up. This helps to keep the hollow in the small of your back ie the best position for your lumbar spine to take the strain and avoid any excess loading.

If you can't kneel into the back of the car, say because there is too high a lip, then load the inside of the car from a side door, and then there is only a short lift – <u>with your head up</u>, to put in the rest of the bags close to the back of the car.

If this is not possible then lift a bag from the trolley in one hand, but lean on the floor of the boot with the other. This gives you another limb to lean on and gets you out of the really bad position of an unsupported bend with extra weight in both hands!

These principles apply to most situations like this eg a visit to the garden centre, or even moving pots in the garden!

The other major rule is don't lift something that is too heavy for you – delegate!

Chair exercises

If your work needs you to spend the large part of the day sitting, then there are a whole host of things that you can do to stop your back and your joints from stiffening up.

As a general concept you need to move around in your chair.

You can:

- shift your weight from one side to the other
- tense one buttock/glute and then the other. Interestingly, people who have recurrent low back pain find it difficult to contract their buttocks individually.

- see if you can move your navel round in a circle, vertically and then horizontally. Try one way and then see if you can do the same going in the other direction.

- hold your hands together with your arms and hands off the desk. Now try and keep your hands still in front of you and rock your pelvis from side to side, without moving your arms or shoulders.

The guideline here is that *any* movement is good. So think about all the movements you *can* do, sitting in your chair. The idea is that you don't spend all day doing this movements. Just a few minutes in every hour.

Rotation of the spine

The spine doesn't just move forwards and back. Don't forget to rotate, or turn the spine as well. It is a very important feature of movement of the body. Almost everything we do has a rotation component. Think how you rotate/turn your arm and hand to bring food to your mouth!

A good example is to turn as far to the left and then to the right when you are sitting and the adverts are on the television!

Stand on one leg for balance and co-ordination

This is one of the simplest ways to improve your balance, co-ordination and even your core stabilising system.

It also works for repeated sprained ankles!

Do this when you are waiting for the kettle to boil, or anything else that means you have to wait for a few minutes like standing in a queue!

All you have to do is put one foot behind the ankle of the other leg and see how long you can stay there.

Start simply with 30secs and gradually build it up. Stand on one leg and then the other, but make sure that you are safe and have something solid to hold onto if you lose your balance.

Shut YOUR eyes

When you get really good at standing on one leg, then try it with your eyes shut.

We rely so much on visual cues as we move around that we can start to lose the amazing feedback system of the body that tells the central processor (brain) where all the bits of us are in space and in relation to each other.

Providing you make sure that you are safe and can stop yourself falling, try getting up from the chair with your eyes closed, and then sit down again. When you can do this easily, and it may take a bit of practice, then you start to trust your other senses and the body will respond. It teaches you "body awareness".

Gradually make the task more difficult. This may be taking a few steps across the room, making sure that there is nothing in the way *before* you close your eyes! You don't have to do much more than this, but repeating it will make a whole range of systems come into play including the body's ability to react more quickly if you feel you are going to fall over.

To swim or not to swim!

It is not actually true that swimming is the very best exercise you can do! If you don't actually like swimming, then don't do it. You will not enjoy it and you will not get any benefit from it. Find an exercise system that you like and enjoy. This might be dancing, martial arts, running, even going to the gym! What is seldom thought of is skipping. This an easy exercise that you can do with very little equipment. Start very simply and gradually build up the time and the effort. After all, there is a good reason why boxers skip so much!

Mattresses

Just a few words here! Most people buy beds from a furniture salesman. They have no medical training and no knowledge of back problems. It is very unlikely that a few moments lying on a bed in a show room is going to tell you whether it is good for your back!

If we are lucky, we will spend a third of our lives in bed! In general, we don't think too much about what, or how the bed is made and we usually buy the bed based on what it looks like and what it costs.

There is a misconception that beds should be hard, if you have a "bad back".

WHAT YOU NEED IS A "SUPPORTIVE" MATTRESS AND NOT THE FLOOR!

To emphasize this point, some years ago when I was working in the NHS, I saw a patient who was complaining of low back pain. He had been sent to the Physiotherapy Department in the hospital by the GP with the advice that he should sleep on a board. He told the GP that he didn't have a board, so it was suggested that he should take a door off in his house and put that on his bed. During the clinical examination of this gentleman, I noticed that he had a significant bruise on his buttock and when I asked him about this he said it was from the door handle that he didn't think to remove before going to bed! So beware the side effects of sleeping on unsuitable surfaces!

Memory foam is excellent, but only if it is of sufficient quality and the right density. If it is cheap, then it probably isn't. Equally, you do not need to spend a huge amount of money on it.

The concept of memory foam is an excellent one in that it allows the bony parts of the body to sink into the mattress, which in turn off loads all the joints of the body. In simple terms, what you need is to lie in bed, on your back, front or either side, with the spine in a neutral position.

Sleep is the time when the body can work to repair itself. If you are uncomfortable in bed at night, then you will toss and turn and the body cannot rest. So take time and good medical advice before deciding which mattress to buy. It is also worth remembering that in general mattresses only last 10 years.

If you look at the picture of this man asleep in bed, you will notice that his upper body and neck are in a flexed position. If he was standing , then his upper body would be leaning forwards. Even though he is lying in this position, he is still putting that bending strain on the spine and he will have an uncomfortable night's sleep. So you really need to look at trying to get into the neutral position to take the load off all the joints. After all, if we are lucky, then we will be spending a third of our lives in bed and we need to be comfortable!

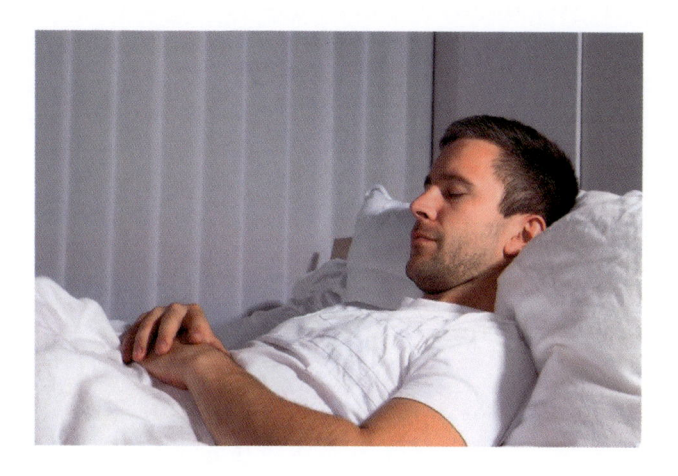

Chapter 12

EXERCISES

There is always a worry that **your** particular condition needs very particular exercises as you progress along the Road to Recovery. This might be flexibility, strength, co-ordination or nerve mobility.

If you are in any doubt about doing exercises then I would ask you to go and see a specialist MSK physiotherapist. This is **our** specialist knowledge.

Doctors can prescribe medication, but they are not trained to prescribe exercises. This is a very important point – it can cause more problems if you do the wrong exercises for your condition – and equally if you do the right exercises wrongly!

HOW TO HELP YOURSELF

There is no doubt that exercise is good for you in many, many ways. Everyone agrees that it is a good thing to do. But what sort of exercise and for what effect? It is an obvious thing to say, but the body is designed to move and if you don't then this will cause problems with the musculo-skeletal system for starters!

With regards to low back pain, we know that the pressures through the lumbar discs, for example, change quite dramatically in different positions. Sitting bolt upright puts the most pressure through the low spine and discs.

Look at your driving position. You should be sitting with the seat about 130 degrees back and with about 3 inches of support for the lumbar spine.

So what position should you be in to do exercises for your back? The simple answer to this is that we expect our bodies to work in all sorts of different positions, so exercise should reflect this. I am not suggesting that you should be doing exercises up a ladder, or with your head stuck underneath the kitchen sink, but you get the idea!

EXERCISES SHOULD BE PAINLESS

If exercises hurt, then don't do them. We advise patients to reduce the exercises if they are hurting, either by the number of repetitions or the range of movement involved. If reducing them in this way reduces the pain, then fine. If not, then speak to your physiotherapist who gave you the exercises and see if there is another way of getting the right result. We work on the basis that it is only the physiotherapist who is allowed to hurt you – you are not allowed to hurt yourself!

It may be that you are doing the exercise incorrectly; you are pushing too hard; you are doing too many repetitions or simply that you are not ready for that exercise.

It is important that you report any pain to your physiotherapist if you are getting an increase in pain while doing any exercises prescribed.

The old adage of "no pain - no gain" is wrong on many levels

Pain often comes on as an indication that tissue damage is about to happen - not necessarily after the damage has been done. It is your nervous system and brain trying to protect you from injury.

Your brain has learnt by experience that certain movements have caused injury and pain and so it will assume that this is what will happen again. The problem is that the brain does not always get it right.

When you are fit and well, there is a smaller gap between when the pain starts and tissue damage begins. But when you suffer an injury, this gap widens and you feel pain well before there is any tissue damage. The reason is that the body is trying to stop you repeating the activity, or movement, that caused the damage.

Under normal circumstance, the body goes through its healing process, the tissues are repaired and the pain stops.

This normal process of pain, inflammation, healing and resolution can sometimes go wrong if the pain continues.

The nervous system and tissues have been "sensitised" and this can happen if there are other factors affecting your body's ability to heal itself. It might be stress caused by the inability to work, or having to look after an elderly relative. All sorts of events can seriously affect the healing rate and prolong the pain. This is a physiological effect.

So it is important to keep a positive attitude and to work with your physiotherapist by carrying out your exercise prescription that supplements the treatment provided. By doing the exercises you are also learning to take responsibility for the future management of the condition. This way you will get the best result in the shortest possible time.

Pain-free exercise is a way of telling your brain that movement is OK and not going to cause you harm

EXERCISES ARE AN ESSENTIAL COMPONENT TO RECOVERY

Correctly prescribed exercises are designed by your physiotherapist to achieve 5 effects for the joints:

FLEXIBILITY

All the joints concerned need to be kept as mobile as possible.

The old adage "If you don't use it, you lose it" applies here!

Or even - **"if you rest - you rust"!**

If you lose the range of movement in the joints then the body simply can't move. It is really so obvious when you think about it!

So flexibility/movement of the joints is the essential starting point to keep everything working well.

STRENGTH

The muscles that work the joints need to be kept as strong as possible. There is no point in having a good range of movement in the joints if the muscles are not strong enough to move them.

There are two essential muscle systems involved:

THE STABILISING SYSTEM.

These are muscles that are working constantly, but at a low intensity level, that work to keep the joint in the best possible position as it moves. They are active components that can contract and keep the right tension around the joint unlike the ligaments which are static "guy ropes" holding the joint together.

There is the *local* stabilising which works very closely to the joints and the *global* stabilising system that works across more than one set of joints to co-ordinate combined joint movements - like walking.

Both these systems are very important and need to be working well, as we very seldom ever use one joint in isolation. With these muscle systems, we need good strength and correct timing for the systems to work efficiently.

THE MOVEMENT SYSTEM

These muscles simply move the joints and need to have all the required strength but working in an integrated and efficient way.

Working individual muscles in the gym will not produce smooth, efficient and integrated movement patterns that the body can and should deliver.

It is one thing to strengthen weak elements in the system and work the cardiovascular system, but it should work alongside individually tailored programmes designed to give you normal patterns of movement that are physiologically correct.

The right movement means efficient movement and takes the load off the joints.

CO-ORDINATION

The muscles and joints have to be trained to work in the way that they were designed, and not in the way that we have adopted due to the way we live and work. Get this aspect right and your life style, work and hobbies become more enjoyable and keeps you fit for longer.

What is often misunderstood is that every movement we do is a co-ordinated effort for the WHOLE body. Even just standing and lifting one arm needs changes in the whole muscle system to make sure that everything is in the right place to take the load shift. Let alone being able to hold the body still and yet allow movement of the arm. It doesn't just happen. The co-ordination of all the muscle and joint system is needed to bring about controlled and efficient movement of the body.

A KEY ELEMENT IS BALANCE

If you have lost balance and co-ordination then you are severely limited in the movements you can achieve.

There are many injuries and disabilities that can result in losing this finely tuned ability of the human being to be able to stand on two feet and then move without falling over.

One of the absolute key elements for balance is the joint movement and fitness of the pelvis with the spine sitting above the pelvis and the hips underneath. The core stabilising muscle system of the trunk certainly needs to be strong but you also need to be able to co-ordinate the movement of the trunk and the pelvis.

About 70% of our patients have problems that involve problems with the spine and pelvis and this is why a large proportion of the exercises in this Recovery Programme focus on restoring the balance and co-ordination of the trunk and pelvis.

We also use them to regain balance and co-ordination for conditions affecting other joints such as knees, feet and even shoulders because problems with these joints will in turn stiffen the spine and pelvis mechanism. This happens because the body is designed to work in a co-ordinated way. Upset one element and the others will start to fail as well.

GENERAL COMMENTS

The problem is that exercises are seldom seen as having any real value.
They are usually viewed as moving parts of the body in a completely boring and time consuming way. So, the average human response is to do some of the exercises while there is still some pain, but to then forget about them when you feel better.

If a doctor prescribes medication for a condition then you are far more likely to take the pills. Exercises work in the same way. There is a huge amount or research, skill and expertise that has been put into a seemingly simple set of exercises.

We have taken into account that we all have busy lives and that few of us can spend an hour a day doing exercises. So the following series of exercises have been specifically devised to provide fast, effective, multi-function activities that, if carried out as "prescribed" will achieve what we all want - resolution of the problem and prevention of any further recurrence.

If you are not sure when to do an exercise programme, try using the time when the adverts are on the television. This way you will be obeying the first rule of rehabilitation exercises "little and often!"

So, don't just sit there through the ads, use the time and move!

The right movement equals efficient movement and takes the load off the joints

A FINAL WORD

I could have written considerably more than I have here, as it is such a huge topic.

I have attempted to write what I think people want to know and in an easy format. I hope I have given those readers enough information that if they want more clinical detail or confirmation of what I have been talking about, then they can search this out for themselves.

I am hopeful that this book offers the right information for people who suffer with low back pain, as well as maybe a different viewpoint for healthcare professionals from all the disciplines that aim to "treat" low back pain.

As I said in the very beginning, it is 7% of patients with low back pain who take up 90% of the costs. If this book helps to stop even a small part of the 93% of patients becoming chronic pain sufferers, then I will have achieved my objective for the patients and maybe some money for the country!

If any reader feels they would like to comment on this book with constructive ideas, questions or observations then I would be very happy to hear your views. The education process is a two way street!

Wendy Emberson MCSP

Printed in Great Britain
by Amazon